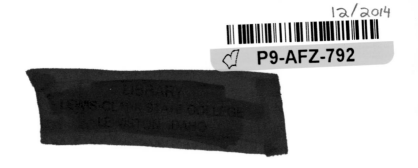

INFECTION CONTROL *for* ADVANCED PRACTICE PROFESSIONALS

Infection Control *for* Advanced Practice Professionals

Edited by
Denise M. Korniewicz, Ph.D., RN, FAAN
Professor & Research Dean
University of North Dakota

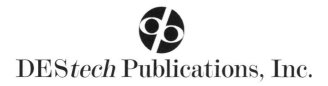

DES*tech* Publications, Inc.

Infection Control for Advanced Practice Professionals

DEStech Publications, Inc.
439 North Duke Street
Lancaster, Pennsylvania 17602 U.S.A.

Printed in the United States of America
10 9 8 7 6 5 4 3 2 1

Main entry under title:
    Infection Control for Advanced Practice Professionals

A DEStech Publications book
Bibliography: p.
Includes index p. 245

Library of Congress Control Number: 2013945041
ISBN No. 978-1-60595-060-0

Contents

Foreword   xi

Preface   xiii

List of Contributors   xv

1. Principles of Infection Control 1
JOAN HEBDEN

1.1. Case Presentation   1
1.2. Essential Content for Infection Control Skills   4
1.3. Creating and Sustaining a Culture of Safety   5
1.4. The Measurement of Performance   6
1.5. Team-led Performance Initiatives   7
1.6. Monitoring and Feedback   9
1.7. Creating an Action Plan for Performance Improvement   12
1.8. Making a Business Case for HAI Prevention   14
1.9. Interpretation/Application of Infection Control Data   14
1.10. Patient Safety and Health System Issues   14
1.11. Summary Points   15
1.12. References   16

2. Safe Infection Control in the Workplace 19
CAROL PATTON and DENISE M. KORNIEWICZ

2.1. Case Presentation   19
2.2. Essential Content for Safe Infection Control
in the Workplace   20
2.3. Employer Standards for Bloodborne Pathogen
Precautions   22
2.4. Personal Protective Equipment (PPE)   23

2.5. Sharps Injuries   27
2.6. Designing Programs of Healthcare Worker Safety   28
2.7. Surveillance and Behavioral-based Performance
     of Healthcare Workers   29
2.8. Creating a Culture of Safe Infection Control Practices   30
2.9. References   31

3. **Patient Safety and the Chain of Infection** **33**
   JOAN HEBDEN
   3.1. Case Presentation   33
   3.2. Essential Content for Infection Control Skills   35
   3.3. Interpretation/Application of Infection Control Data   44
   3.4. Patient Safety and Health System: Infection
        Control Practices   45
   3.5. Summary Points   46
   3.6. References   46

4. **Essentials of Epidemiologic Measures and
   Data Interpretation** **49**
   MAHER M. EL-MASRI and DAVY TAWADROUS
   4.1. Case Presentation   49
   4.2. Measures of Disease Frequency   50
   4.3. Measures of Disease-exposure Association   55
   4.4. Statistical Probability (*P*. Value)   61
   4.5. Clinical Versus Statistical Significance   66
   4.6. Summary Points   67
   4.7. References   67

5. **Infection Control in Acute Care Settings** **69**
   JEANNE HINTON SIEGEL
   5.1. Case Presentation   69
   5.2. Essential Content for Infection Control   72
   5.3. Hand Hygiene   75
   5.4. Engineering Controls   78
   5.5. New Monitoring Techniques   80
   5.6. Use of Isolation to Prevent the Spread of Infections   83
   5.7. Review of Healthcare Environments   86
   5.8. Advanced Practice Professionals' Roles in
        Public Health   89
   5.9. References   91

6. Infection Control in Critical Care Settings 95
MARY WYCKOFF

6.1. Case Presentation   95
6.2. Essential Content for Infection Control   96
6.3. Hospital Acquired Infections in Critical Care   97
6.4. Attributable Cost of Hospital Acquired Infections   98
6.5. How to Effectively Process Change   100
6.6. Conclusion and Summary Points   106
6.7. References   107

7. Infection Control in the Emergency Department Settings 109
MICHELLE WRIGHT

7.1. Case Presentation   109
7.2. Essential Content for Infection Control Skills   112
7.3. Precautions   113
7.4. Unknown Illness   113
7.5. Biochemical Agents   117
7.6. Trauma   118
7.7. Travel   119
7.8. Equipment Sharing   120
7.9. Patient Mobility   121
7.10. Overcrowding   122
7.11. Empirical Antibiotic Therapy   122
7.12. Novel Approaches   123
7.13. Summary Points   124
7.14. References   124

8. Infection Control in Primary Care Settings. 126
CAROL PATTON and DENISE M. KORNIEWICZ

8.1. Case Presentation   129
8.2. Essential Content for Infection Control Skills   130
8.3. Creating the Culture of Infection Control in Primary Care Settings   131
8.4. Strategies for Best Practices for Infection Control in Primary Care Settings   132
8.5. Summary Points   139
8.6. References   139

9. Infection Control Principles for Long-term Care Environments 141

JUDITH SELTZER and DENISE M. KORNIEWICZ

9.1. Case Presentation   141
9.2. Essential Content for Infection Control Skills   143
9.3. General Environmental Issues (Wheelchairs, Hand Rails, Walkers, Cleaning Rooms)   152
9.4. Regulatory Measures   153
9.5. Summary Points   153
9.6. References   155

10. Infection Control in the Home 157

JEANETTE ADAMS

10.1. Case Presentation   157
10.2. Essential Content for Infection Control Skills   159
10.3. Health Care Providers   163
10.4. Multidrug-Resistant Organisms   165
10.5. Interpretation/Application of Infection Control Data   165
10.6. Discussion about Patient Safety and Health System Issues Related to ICP   166
10.7. Summary Points   167
10.8. References   168

11. Infection Control Practice in Mental Health Settings 171

JAMES WEIDEL

11.1. Case Presentation   171
11.2. Environment of Care of the Psychiatric/Mental Health Facility   174
11.3. Limited Access to Supplies   175
11.4. Linen and Clothing   176
11.5. Provider-Patient Interaction   176
11.6. Food Safety   177
11.7. Patient Handling of Food   179
11.8. Sanitation and Housekeeping   180
11.9. Risk Factors Associated with Infection Among Psychiatric Patients   180
11.10. Isolation   182
11.11. Transmission Based Precautions   183

11.12. Restraints and Infection Control   184
11.13. Conclusion   186
11.14. Summary Points   186
11.15. References   187

12. Infection Control in Ambulatory Surgical Centers. . . .189
JUDITH SELTZER

12.1. Case Presentation   189
12.2. Essential Content for Infection Control in
    Ambulatory Surgical Settings   191
12.3. Regulatory Influences   192
12.4. Infection Control Monitoring   198
12.5. Active Participation   199
12.6. Long-term Infection Control Principles in
    Ambulatory Surgical Settings   200
12.7. Summary Points   201
12.8. References   203

13. Infection Control in the Community 205
JEANETTE ADAMS

13.1. Case Presentation   205
13.2. Essential Content for Infection Control Skills   206
13.3. Food Borne Infections   206
13.4. Prevention of Infectious Diseases   208
13.5. Methicillin Resistant Staphylococcus Aureus (MRSA)   210
13.6. *Clostridium Difficile* (C-diff.)   211
13.7. Human Immunodeficiency Virus (HIV)   211
13.8. Interpretation/Application of Infection Control Data   212
13.9. Discussion about Patient Safety and Health System
    Issues Related To ICP   212
13.10. Summary Points   213
13.11. References   213

14. Infection Control for Emergency Mobile
Health Units 215
MICHELLE WRIGHT

14.1. Case Presentation   215
14.2. Essential Content for Infection Control Skills   217
14.3. Vector Borne Illnesses   221
14.4. Overcrowding   224

14.5. Personnel Safety   225

14.6. Medically Trained Volunteers   226

14.7. Untrained Volunteers   227

14.8. Interpretation/Application of Infection Control Data   228

14.9. Patient Safety and Health System Issues   228

14.10. Summary Points   230

14.11. References   231

15. Future Issues in Monitoring for Safe Infection
Control Practices 233
DENISE M. KORNIEWICZ

15.1. Case Presentation   233

15.2. Essential Content Infection Control of the Future   234

15.3. Future Engineering Controls   237

15.4. Safety Through Knowledge   239

15.5. Future Patient Participation, Public Awareness and
          Patient Advocacy   242

15.6. Summary Points   243

15.7. References   244

Index   245

Foreword

At last is published a long-needed text for advanced practice nurses (APNs), providing them with the information essential to the care of essentially every patient they will encounter. Infection Control for Advanced Practice Professionals fills a void in the literature and recognizes the importance of a team approach to the prevention of infections in the variety of care settings in which APNs are practicing. The book is particularly timely and relevant because it appropriately places infection prevention solidly within the larger patient safety movement and affirms that preventing infections is *everybody's* concern. In acute care settings, for example, infection control has occasionally been relegated to the infection prevention specialist (e.g., infection control nurse or hospital epidemiologist) or the infection control committee. This has shown to be ineffective in any setting. It is those who 'touch' the patients and oversee their care who must assume the responsibility for preventing untoward events such as infections. While not all infections are preventable, there is indeed room for improvement. This comprehensive reference is a first and essential step in that direction!

ELAINE LARSON, RN, PhD, FAAN, CIC
Professor of Pharmaceutical and Therapeutic Research
Associate Dean for Research
School of Nursing
Professor of Epidemiology
Joseph Mailman School of Public Health
Columbia University
Editor, American Journal of Infection Control

Preface

Infection Control for Advanced Practice Professionals is the result of years of research during which the author has attempted to combine clinical research about infection control with essential information needed by advanced practice professionals. Advanced practice professionals such as nurse practitioners, clinical nurse specialists, nurse midwives, physical therapists, physician assistants or other mid-level healthcare providers need to be aware of infection control practices since they are often the first person that is contacted by a patient. The advanced practice practitioner has general knowledge about emerging infections but often has little experience with the specific content associated with the basic and advanced concepts of infection control. The purpose of this book is to provide the essential content about infection control for advanced practice professionals so that they can determine the best practices needed for treatment options.

Much has been written about infection control; however, what has not been written has been a practical approach to infection control content for a variety of clinical and non-clinical settings. The book has been divided into four major themes that mirror the important concepts associated with infection control across a variety of settings. The four areas include: (1) general principles of infection control (safe practices, chain of infection, interpreting data); (2) patients in traditional clinical settings (workplace, hospital, emergency rooms); (3) patients from alternate settings (home, mental health, ambulatory or surgical clinics); and (4) patients in global health settings (community, mobile units, future monitoring).

A unique feature of this book is the integration and use of a "case study" related to the topic for each chapter. This feature attempts to provide the reader with the critical decision making skills needed for safe and effective clinical practice. Often, advanced practice professionals are the only healthcare provider available, and their ability to logically and methodically make a diagnosis is dependent on their critical thinking and clinical skills. This book provides a practical approach to the principles of infection control practices while systematically providing the reader with the content needed about similar patients who may present in similar clinical or non-clinical settings.

The author's deep gratitude is expressed to all the chapter authors who provided essential content for the book. Thanks go to the numerous friends and colleagues who facilitated this effort. A special thanks is given to my research associate, Michelle Wright, who worked diligently on editing each chapter's content. Others who assisted me with the initial development of the content include Dr. Laurel Shepherd and Dr. Joanne Duffy. Finally, deepest appreciation to my sister, Sandy Korniewicz, who patiently provided encouragement to complete the project, and my adopted sister, Margaret Brack, whose positive support helped me to successfully complete this endeavor.

DENISE M. KORNIEWICZ

List of Contributors

JEANETTE ADAMS, Ph.D., RN, ACNS-BC, CRNI
College of Nursing
University of North Dakota
Grand Forks, North Dakota, USA

MAHER M. EL-MASRI, Ph.D., RN
Faculty of Nursing
University of Windsor
Windsor, Ontario, Canada

JOAN N. HEBDEN, RN, MS, CIC
Wolters Kluwer Health – Sentri7
Bellevue, Washington, USA

CAROL M. PATTON, DrPH., RN, FNP-BC, CRNP, CNE
College of Nursing & Health Professions
Drexel University
Philadelphia, PA, USA

JUDITH A. SELTZER, MS., BSN, BN, CNOR
Surgical Clinical Director, Corporate Accounts
Molnlycke Health Care
Norcross, Georgia, USA

JEANNE H. SIEGEL, Ph.D., ARNP
School of Nursing and Health Science
University of Miami
Miami, Florida, USA

DAVY TAWADROUS, BHSc, MD(c)
Schulich School of Medicine
Western University
London, Ontario, Canada

JAMES J. WEIDEL, MSN, RN
College of Nursing and Health Sciences
Florida International University
Boca Raton, Florida, USA

MICHELLE L. WRIGHT, MS, RN
College of Nursing
University of North Dakota
Grand Forks, North Dakota, USA

MARY WYCKOFF, Ph.D.
University of California, Davis
Sacramento, California, USA

CHAPTER 1

Principles of Infection Control

JOAN HEBDEN RN, MS, CIC

This chapter will present a basic case study that will include the current perspectives of infection control as well as major statistics associated with the increased numbers of healthcare associated infections (HAIs) or community acquired infections. Emphasis will be targeted to the advanced practice healthcare professional.

1.1. CASE PRESENTATION

Anne is a nurse practitioner who has recently been hired as a team member to provide care to patients requiring a variety of cardiac surgical interventions at a major academic medical center. The hospital performs more than 1,000 cardiothoracic surgeries annually and is designated as a Magnet™ Hospital. During the hospital orientation, Anne learns from the Chief Medical Officer (CMO) that the facility has a strategic goal to achieve designation as a top performing hospital for quality. The CMO states that patient safety is the number one priority for the organization with emphasis on the prevention of healthcare-associated infections (HAIs). As part of the strategic plan to promote a culture of safety and individual accountability, multidisciplinary teams focused on the translation of evidence-based practices at the bedside are being implemented by each clinical department. The message from senior leadership to Anne was to deliver high quality, cost-effective care at each and every patient encounter.

Prior to beginning her patient care duties, Anne met with Dr. Thomas, the Chief of Cardiac Surgery, who asked her to serve on the department's quality and safety committee. A report card displaying multiple quality metrics with a data dictionary and target goals for the department was presented to her. The process metrics included: compliance with hand hygiene, best practices for the insertion of central venous catheters, discontinuation of urinary catheters within 24 hours after surgery and elevation of the head of the bed 30 degrees for ventilated patients. Outcome measures included: central line-associated bloodstream infections (CLABSI), catheter-associated urinary tract infections (CA-UTI), and post-operative mediastinitis occurring in coronary artery bypass graft (CABG) patients. Also included were some of the surgical care improvement project (SCIP) infection measures, specifically prophylactic antibiotics received within 60 minutes prior to surgical incision, appropriate selection of prophylactic antibiotic, and discontinuation of the prophylactic antibiotic within 48 hours after cardiac surgery end time. Dr. Thomas informed Anne that she will have several collaborative partners to work with her on achieving the target goals for each quality metric: Beth, a senior nurse on the cardiothoracic step-down unit; Dr. Miller, a fellow on the cardiac surgery team; Dr. Jones, an anesthesiologist; Cindy, a quality improvement coordinator; Michele, an infection preventionist, and John, the service line director for Cardiac Surgery.

At the end of the meeting, Dr. Thomas remarked that achieving recognition as a top performer in the provision of safe patient care is extremely important to the department due to recent incorporation of performance measures into the financial reimbursement systems and the transparency of institutional HAI rates on public report cards. Of particular concern to the department is performance related to hand hygiene compliance, a recent increase in the rate of post-operative mediastinitis among CABG patients and the rate of CLABSI occurring in patients in the Cardiothoracic Intensive Care Unit (CTICU).

Anne is assigned to the cardiothoracic step-down unit, a 35-bed unit caring for both pre-operative patients requiring inpatient care prior to their cardiac surgery as well as post-operative patients discharged from the CTICU. Anne's patient care duties include rounding with the surgical team in the early morning to address patient issues that may have arisen during the night and to check the results of blood work and again in the late afternoon to assess deposition of each patient. During rounds, Anne has the opportunity to observe the teams' compliance with several infection prevention and control practices that relate to poor performance on departmental quality metrics. Although alcohol hand sanitizing products are readily available outside of the patient rooms along with visible signage encouraging hand hygiene before and after each patient contact, not all the care providers perform the activity. When one of the surgeons fails to use the sanitizer, Anne picks up the product and offers it to the physician. The surgeon uses the product and thanks Anne for the reminder. Later that day, one of the nursing staff compliments Anne for her commitment to improving hand hygiene compliance and remarks, "everyone has seen this surgeon be noncompliant, but no one felt comfortable pointing it out".

One day during rounds, Michele, the infection preventionist, participates to discuss a positive blood culture result for *Klebsiella pneumoniae* in a post-operative patient. The patient was discharged from the CTICU two days prior to the positive blood culture with a central venous catheter in place. Michele queried the team regarding a possible source of the bacteremia and inquired about the need for central venous access on the step-down unit. She informed the team that a CLABSI that develops within 2 calendar days of transfer from the CTICU would be attributable to the ICU. The cardiac surgery fellow tells Michele that this is a primary bloodstream infection related to the central line and an order would be placed for line removal. The fellow also notes that the central line was no longer needed to care for this patient and should have been discontinued when the patient arrived on the step-down unit. Anne suggests that for new patients with a central line, an assessment of the necessity of the line be performed during the admission process and included as part of daily rounds.

After being on the unit for several weeks, Anne has cared for a couple of patients who have required readmission for post-operative mediastinitis following a CABG procedure. She recalls that the rate of mediastinitis had increased in the last quarter to 1.5% from 0.2% and 0.4% in the prior two quarters. The Office of Risk Management for the organization notifies the departmental quality team members that one of these patients has obtained legal counsel and a lawsuit is anticipated. The risk management representative requests that a quality of care review be conducted to determine if any violations to the standard of care occurred. The review is coordinated by the quality improvement coordinator who identifies that this patient did not perform a pre-operative shower with chlorhexidine skin antiseptic and although the appropriate prophylactic antibiotic was chosen, the drug was not administered until after the incision was made. A meeting of the quality team is convened to review all recent cases of mediastinitis to further identify performance improvement opportunities.

1.2. ESSENTIAL CONTENT FOR INFECTION CONTROL SKILLS

Healthcare-associated infections (HAIs) are a common cause of patient morbidity and mortality in the United States. The Centers for Disease Control and Prevention (CDC) estimates approximately 2 million HAIs associated with nearly 100,000 deaths occur annually among hospitalized patients. In the past decade, HAIs have been pushed to the forefront as a national patient safety initiative, since the publication of the Institute of Medicine's report, To Err is Human, which drew attention to HAIs as "preventable harms". Consumer advocacy groups, legislative bodies and accreditation organizations served as catalysts for hospitals to allocate money and resources to infection control programs. As of January 2012, 28 states have passed legislation that require public reporting of one or more HAIs with 23 of those states stipulating the use of the National Healthcare Safety Network (NHSN). The public reporting of HAI outcome data for inter-hospital comparisons and consumer choice carries a reputational risk for hospitals. Additionally, economic risk exists from the pay-for-performance reform enacted by Congress through the Centers for Medicare and Medicaid Services (CMS).

Through the Affordable Care Act Value Based purchasing program, CMS now requires national public reporting of CLABSI, CA-UTI surgical site infections (SSI) associated with colon procedures and abdominal hysterectomies through the NHSN, and additional HAIs are anticipated to follow. Historically, HAIs resulted in additional reimbursement by the payment systems. However, with recent reports demonstrating that many HAIs are preventable, payors will be paying "less". The financial benefit of HAI reduction is estimated to be $25 billion to $31.5 billion in medical cost savings (Scott, 2009).

A 2010 white paper entitled "Moving Toward Elimination of Healthcare-Associated Infections: A Call to Action" provides a framework for achieving what was once thought of as an improbable goal (Cardo, 2010). To be successful, the perception that HAIs are unavoidable consequences of complex medical care must be replaced with a patient safety mindset that each and every one of these occurrences is *avoidable* and *unacceptable*. The pillars of this framework include: implementing evidence-based practices that protect patients; aligning incentives to promote system-wide strategies for HAI prevention; addressing gaps in knowledge through research; and collecting data to target prevention efforts and to measure progress. Several suggested strategies to increase adherence to evidence-based practice guidelines include senior leadership support, education and engagement of the bedside clinicians, empowerment of the front-line staff to intercede on behalf of patient safety and feedback of HAI data in a timely fashion to the clinicians. This chapter will focus on two major paradigm shifts occurring in the field of infection control. First, the responsibility to reduce HAIs has shifted from the members of the infection control program to the multidisciplinary team providing bedside care with input from the infection control experts. Advanced practice nurses will have a critical role by promoting collaborative practice utilizing evidence-based standards of care, encouraging a spirit of inquiry and being strong patient advocates. Second, the shift from perceiving HAIs as unavoidable consequences of complex medical care with no impact on the financial bottom line to a mindset of targeting zero HAIs to avoid financial penalties. Perencevich and colleagues eloquently entitled their 2007 Society for Healthcare Epidemiology of America (SHEA) guideline, "Raising Standards While Watching the Bottom Line: Making a Business Case for Infection Control" (Perencevich, 2007).

1.3. CREATING AND SUSTAINING A CULTURE OF SAFETY

When Anne arrives at her new job, the CMO of the organization is visible at orientation with the message that patient safety is a top strategic priority with particular emphasis on the prevention of HAIs . . .

The National Quality Forum Safe Practices for Better Healthcare-2010 Update: A Consensus Report details 34 practices that have been identified as effective in reducing adverse outcomes of healthcare. These practices are organized into seven functional categories with a culture of safety built on organizational awareness of performance gaps, measurement and feedback to leadership and staff and team-led performance improvement initiatives leading the list. The prevention of HAIs is a distinct functional category with the following identified safe practices: CLABSI prevention, SSI prevention, care of the ventilated patient, multi-drug-resistant organism prevention, and CA-UTI prevention. In order to drive the best practices for prevention of HAIs to the bedside, leadership endorsement and support is critical. The goal is to instill a proactive approach to quality patient care rather than a reactive strategy that leads to short-lived results.

1.4. THE MEASUREMENT OF PERFORMANCE

Anne meets with Dr. Thomas, the Chief of Cardiac Surgery, who asks her to serve on the departmental quality and safety committee. A report card displaying multiple quality metrics with a data dictionary and target goals is shared with her . . .

The elevation of awareness of the gaps in quality infection performance metrics to the frontline staff is essential to the success of improvement initiatives. However, the staff need to understand how the data were collected to establish clinical credibility and to know the expectations related to their role in the prevention of HAI. The quality metrics included on the case study report card are representative of a measurement strategy that includes mandated SCIP and the Joint Commission process measures as well as HAI outcome measures chosen for local, state or national public reporting. As noted by Streed in a recent American Journal of Infection Control (AJIC) practice forum (Streed, 2011), process measures tend to be more objective and dichotomous in nature, hence removing the potential for inter-rater bias that may exist with the use of NHSN HAI surveillance definitions. An important component of a quality report card is a data dictionary that defines the metrics. The SCIP process measure of compliance with the administration of surgical prophylaxis defines "within one hour of the incision" and can be answered as either "yes" or "no". The metric is reported as a percent by dividing the number of compliant episodes by the number of selected surgical procedures.

The Joint Commission National Patient Safety Goal 07.01.01 requires hospitals to comply with either the current CDC or World Health Organization's hand hygiene guidelines, which stipulate monitoring of compliance with feedback of data. The method of monitoring is not prescriptive and may be based on the definition criteria of state-led collaboratives. Generally, hand hygiene compliance data is based on "secret shopper" observations either upon entry or exit from the patient room (or both) and the metric is reported as a percent by dividing the number of compliant observations by the number of hand hygiene opportunities.

The calculation of the HAI outcome rates for CLABSI, CA-UTI and

TABLE 1.1. Calculating Device-Associated and Procedure-Associated Infection Rates.

Device-associated Infection Rate = $$\frac{\text{Number of device-associated infections for an infection site}}{\text{Number of device-days}} \times 1000$$
Example: Central Line-associated BSI Rate per 1000 Central Line-days = $$\frac{\text{Number of central line-associated BSI}}{\text{Number of central line-days}} \times 1000$$
Procedure-associated Infection Rate = $$\frac{\text{Number of procedure-associated infections for a particular procedure}}{\text{Number of procedures}} \times 1$$
Example: Surgical Site Infection (SSI) Associated with Hysterectomy Procedures

ventilator-associated pneumonia (VAP) as defined by NHSN is determined by dividing the number of device-associated infections that meet standardized definitions by the number of device days and multiplying by 1000. SSI rates are calculated by dividing the number of SSIs by the number of specific operative procedures and multiplying the results by 100 (Table 1.1). SSI rates can be stratified by risk index based on the presence of specific patient risk factors.

The quantification of these quality metrics in a valid and meaningful way is necessary to promote understanding and ownership of the data by the frontline staff who are responsible for executing the best practices for HAI prevention. Gurses and colleagues (2008) conducted a qualitative study in two surgical ICUs to assess compliance with HAI evidence-based practice guidelines. The authors found that the presentation of CLABSI data as a rate per 1,000 central line days—4.6/1,000 line days with a target of < 4.0/1,000 line days—was not particularly relevant to the nurses and defined it as "expectation ambiguity". As a result of this finding, the data was communicated as a raw number of CLABSIs. The authors emphasize that attention to behavioral factors is critical for assessing the "readiness" of the staff to consider alternative processes of care.

1.5. TEAM-LED PERFORMANCE INITIATIVES

Mutidisciplinary teams focused on the translation of evidence-based practices to the bedside are being implemented by departments. Dr. Thomas informs Anne that she will have several collaborative partners . . .

A resounding message from organizations committed to improving the safety of healthcare delivery is to create a quality infrastructure that engages team-led performance improvement interventions. Teamwork promotes a standardized approach to patient care. An endorsement for this approach is described by Peter Pronovost, M.D., Ph.D.: "There's a large potential to reduce infections by simplifying the process into three things: standardize what you do, create independent checks for known processes and when things go wrong, learn from them". Pronovost and colleagues (2006) tested the efficacy of a checklist of five evidence-based practices culled from lengthy guidelines for the prevention of CLABSI in a large ICU cohort study throughout Michigan, known as the Keystone Project. The use of the intervention bundle, which focused on hand hygiene, use of full sterile barrier precautions, skin antisepsis with chlorhexidine, avoiding femoral line placements and removal of unnecessary catheters, resulted in a substantial and sustained reduction in CLABSI rates. An important operational concept in this study was the designation of a physician and nurse champion in each of the ICUs to facilitate the implementation of the CLABSI bundle by the bedside staff. A key finding from culture surveys administered in each of the participating ICUs was that the highest percentage of ICUs sustaining zero CLABSIs for 5 or more months were associated with the highest percentage of respondents reporting a good teamwork climate (Figure 1.1).

Although it would seem that teamwork, which is associated with effective communication and a shared mental model of the task at hand, would be hardwired into the field of healthcare, data from the Joint Commission suggests that communication breakdowns are frequently the root cause of adverse outcomes of care. The development of collaborative partnerships among healthcare providers is an evolving mindset. To assist healthcare professionals in this journey, the Agency for Healthcare Research and Quality (AHRQ) developed the system Team STEPPS (Strategies and Tools to Enhance Performance and Patient Safety). One critical component of teamwork that this system addresses is increasing team awareness and clarifying team roles and responsibilities. Transitioning from traditional work processes—"that is how it has always been done"—to redesigned systems of care is a major challenge in the translation of evidence-based practices to the bedside. Utilizing the concept of a "dress rehearsal" which involves mentally mapping and physically walking through each new practice allows for the identification of breakdowns in compliance and can preemptively mitigate concerns about compatibility with existing workflow patterns (Figure 1.2).

The rehearsal may identify the need for additional supplies and resources. Therefore, it is useful to have a financial representative on the team who can assist with the economic evaluation of the intervention.

1.6. MONITORING AND FEEDBACK

The message from senior leadership to Anne and the other clinicians was to deliver high quality, cost-effective care with each and every patient encounter. During rounds, when one of the surgeons fails to use the hand sanitizer, Anne reminds him. One of the nurses remarks "everyone has seen this surgeon be noncompliant with hand hygiene, but no one felt comfortable pointing it out".

In order to obtain high standards of practice every time for every patient, the processes of care need to be monitored and feedback provided regarding practice violations. Accountability auditing can detect individuals, processes or outcomes contributing to less than optimal performance. The example of noncompliance with hand hygiene by

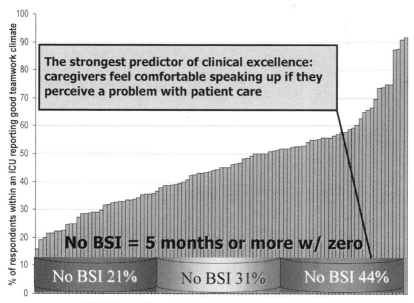

FIGURE 1.1. Teamwork climate across Michigan ICUs.

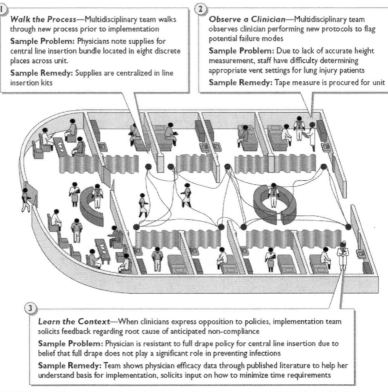

① **Walk the Process**—Multidisciplinary team walks through new process prior to implementation

Sample Problem: Physicians note supplies for central line insertion bundle located in eight discrete places across unit.

Sample Remedy: Supplies are centralized in line insertion kits

② **Observe a Clinician**—Multidisciplinary team observes clinician performing new protocols to flag potential failure modes

Sample Problem: Due to lack of accurate height measurement, staff have difficulty determining appropriate vent settings for lung injury patients

Sample Remedy: Tape measure is procured for unit

③ **Learn the Context**—When clinicians express opposition to policies, implementation team solicits feedback regarding root cause of anticipated non-compliance

Sample Problem: Physician is resistant to full drape policy for central line insertion due to belief that full drape does not play a significant role in preventing infections

Sample Remedy: Team shows physician efficacy data through published literature to help her understand basis for implementation, solicits input on how to minimize time requirements

FIGURE 1.2. The advisory board concept of a "dress rehersal". Published in their report, Putting Perfection into Action—originally presented by the Advisory Board's Nursing Executive Center, 2007.

the surgeon in the case study illustrates how staff empowerment in ensuring best practices can lead to real-time feedback without retribution. When accountability is enforced by your team members who have embraced a zero tolerance for violations, the processes become hardwired into the unit culture. Preas and colleagues at the University of Maryland Medical Center (2011) reported on the use of a dedicated nurse champion with responsibility to monitor and provide real time feedback to surgical ICU staff regarding compliance with infection control measures. The unit successfully reduced the rate of CLABSI from the NHSN 90th percentile to zero which was sustained for many months.

Process measures that have target goals of 100% compliance can be monitored during clinical rounds or through manual or automated surveillance methods. As suggested in the case study, the assessment of central line necessity can become a standard question during team rounds. Other process measures that are part of HAI prevention bundles, such as head of the bed elevation 30 degrees for ventilated patients, maintaining the urinary catheter drainage bag below the level of the bladder, and maintaining a dry and intact dressing on central line sites can be efficiently monitored during patient encounters. The tracking of the SCIP process measures is usually performed by the quality improvement staff through manual chart review or by utilizing automated surveillance with data stratified by department, surgeon and anesthesiologist. Prompt feedback to the individual care provider about cases that did not meet the performance standard can mitigate future occurrences. The attention to process measure compliance can be raised by posting graphic displays of data in common areas of the unit and sharing the data at organizational and unit-level quality forums. The question at these forums should be, "How are we doing—did we reach every patient"? Several organizations, such as the Leapfrog Group and the Hospital Quality Alliance, have collected data through voluntary reporting of HAI process measures which allows hospitals to externally benchmark their progress against other hospitals.

The collection of HAI outcome data is in the purview of the infection prevention program. The infection preventionists (IPs) conduct active, prospective surveillance for HAIs utilizing standardized NHSN definitions and case-finding methods. The performance of surveillance is considered the most important data management activity of infection control programs (Scheckler, 1998). Focus is generally on device-associated and procedure-associated HAIs, as these infections are linked to potentially modifiable risk factors and have been chosen as reportable conditions at the state and federal level. Importantly, the standardization of surveillance methods allows for prompt identification of adverse trends. As with HAI process measures, the production of meaningful and accessible data reports for key stakeholders is an essential feedback mechanism. These reports can be used to internally display the rates of multiple units' data for easy recognition of best and poorest performance units and can stimulate communication among units (Figure 1.3).

The best performance units, or the "positive deviants", can share their performance improvement strategies with their colleagues. Positive deviance— building on the capabilities people already have to solve a problem rather than telling them how to change—found its way into healthcare with a regional healthcare initiative in Pittsburgh focused on improving hand hygiene. The idea of finding solutions from insiders

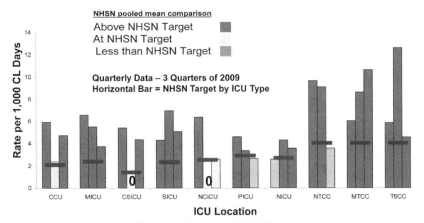

FIGURE 1.3. *ICU central-line associated BSI rates—by quarter.*

had originated with Jerry Sternin, a Tufts University nutritionist who, along with his wife, used the approach with overwhelming success to address the problem of malnutrition in Vietnam (Gawande, 2007). Additionally, these reports can tell the story of the organization's journey to eliminating HAIs to accrediting agencies, which have as a programmatic requirement, an infection prevention risk assessment with prioritization of reduction efforts.

1.7. CREATING AN ACTION PLAN FOR PERFORMANCE IMPROVEMENT

After being on the unit for several weeks, Anne has cared for a couple of patients who have required readmission for postoperative mediastinitis following a CABG procedure. She recalls that the rate of mediastinitis had increased in the last quarter to 1.5% from 0.2% and 0.4% in the prior two quarters . . .

The reported rate of mediastinitis SSIs following CABG surgery ranges from 0.12% to 5% with an associated mortality as high as 40% (Kohut, 2011). Perencevich and colleagues (2007) cite a mean excess length of stay of 25.7 days and a mean attributable cost of $17,944 to CABG-associated SSI. In light of the significant morbidity and mortality associated with this organ space infection, an increase in mediastinitis warrants further investigation. In the case study example, a quality meeting is convened to review recent cases of infection with the knowledge that at least one of the cases did not meet best practice for pre-operative showering and the timing of antibiotic prophylaxis. Prior to the meeting, Anne reviews SSI process and outcome data with Cindy, the quality improvement coordinator, and Michele, the infection preventionist. The Cardiac Surgery Department SCIP measured data reveals excellent compliance with the exception of the timing of antibiotic prophylaxis within 60 minutes of incision, which had fallen to 93% in the previous six months. A metric for patient compliance with pre-operative showering, on the pre-operative checklist as a yes or no answer, is not available. The mediastinitis rate of 1.5% is based on 3 cases of infection divided by 195 CABG procedures, which is the average number of procedures per quarter performed over the prior 24 months. A review of pathogen data and surgeon-specific rates of infection does not suggest a common organism or surgeon associated with the infections. However, a commonality among the cases for this quarter as well as the prior two quarters is poor patient compliance with pre-operative showering and practice violations with the timing of antibiotic prophylaxis.

At the multidisciplinary quality forum, the team reviews the current care processes for educating patients regarding pre-operative showering with chlorhexidine and the administration of antibiotic prophylaxis. Written instructions for preoperative showering along with chlorhexidine soap packets are provided to the patients during their preoperative visit with approximately 20% of the elective surgical patients having their preoperative visit in the surgeons' office. The compliance with the provision of showering instructions to the patients is not known. Antibiotic prophylaxis is under the purview of the anesthesia staff and is generally administered in the Operating Room. Cefazolin is administered as an intravenous push medication except to those patients reporting allergies to penicillins or beta-lactams or a history of MRSA. In these cases, Vancomycin is the appropriate alternative but requires that administration begin 60–120 minutes before the incision. A review of the case data determines that the recent mediastinitis cases received Vancomycin prophylaxis. The team members develop an action plan with the following items: (1) perform a compliance audit related to the provision of preoperative showering instructions to elective CABG patients; (2) contact the Information Technology Group regarding the creation of an automated report to monitor patient response to the question of preoperative showering on the preoperative checklist; and (3) evaluate the management of patients requiring Vancomycin prophylaxis to ensure timely administration.

1.8. MAKING A BUSINESS CASE FOR HAI PREVENTION

The development of HAI reduction action plans may require additional resources, equipment or work redesign. One approach to creating a compelling business case to justify these action plans is to calculate cost-savings obtained by avoiding infections using attributable cost estimates. Another approach is to focus on the potential gains in revenue associated with HAI reduction. As patients without HAIs are discharged sooner from the hospital, the available bed-days for new patients increase, thereby increasing volumes and revenue. As an example: the CABG SSI mean excess length of stay (LOS) is 26 days, therefore, preventing 10 CABG SSIs would open up 260 bed-days. If the average LOS without complication is 4 days, then 65 new patients can be admitted. Along with these approaches, the impact of limited reimbursement by CMS for complications of specific HAIs along with readmission penalties will provide additional financial incentives for administrators to fund HAI reduction interventions.

1.9. INTERPRETATION/APPLICATION OF INFECTION CONTROL DATA

Advanced practice nurses (APNs) have a unique skill set to offer as members of the multidisciplinary teams assigned to lead HAI reduction initiatives. As autonomous, expert clinicians, they are key stakeholders in the quality of care that is provided to the patients they serve. APNs are a constant presence in the clinical environment and become intimately familiar with the work system as well as the behavioral patterns of the care providers. By fostering the communication of best practices for HAI prevention through role modeling, education and multidisciplinary collaboration, APNs contribute significantly to a culture of patient safety.

1.10. PATIENT SAFETY AND HEALTH SYSTEM ISSUES

The increased attention to patient safety in healthcare facilities has been driven by regulatory agencies, advocacy groups, litigators and most importantly, the patients' themselves. This attention has been welcomed by infection prevention and control professionals who focus on the improvement of patient safety through HAI reduction. Historically, many IPs were solo practitioners, serving as data collectors and disseminators, and "policing" the practice of clinicians when infection rates were deemed too high. In the last decade, these professionals have learned to be collaborative partners with the "real" infection preventionists—the clinicians and their support staff who deliver hands-on care to patients. The translation of evidence-based practices to the bedside requires flexibility to change traditional ways of practice, clarification about the role and responsibilities of each individual and empowerment of each person to hold others accountable without fear of retribution. The identification of clinical champions, such as APNs, establishes a liaison for the IP staff who can assist with identification of barriers to adherence with evidence-based practices.

The oversight of infection control practices within hospitals has now extended to payors and consumers with the public reporting of HAI process and outcome metrics. Pay-for-performance reform and consumer choice will directly impact the revenue stream of hospitals. The potential financial consequences and reputational risk associated with poor performance metrics will catalyze the development of care systems that are prevention-oriented. Last, the launching of the Partnership for Patients by the Department of Health and Human Services, with the aggressive goals of decreasing preventable hospital-acquired conditions by 40% and hospital readmissions by 20% by the end of 2013, will challenge healthcare organizations to examine their current acute care-based prevention strategies, discharge planning processes and patient education programs. A national collaborative of this magnitude speaks loudly and clearly that patient safety is non-negotiable.

1.11. SUMMARY POINTS

- HAIs are considered to be "preventable harms".
- The consistent and sustained translation of evidence-based practices to the bedside requires a culture of organizational and personal accountability.
- Team-led performance improvement interventions foster interconnectedness in prevention efforts among key stakeholders.
- Monitoring performance with verbal and visual feedback of data will assist with hardwiring key processes of care.
- The economic impact of HAIs should be quantified to build a business case for infection prevention.

1.12. REFERENCES

Advisory Board Company. (2007) Case profile of Keystone ICU Collaborative (Michigan Hospital Association). *Putting Perfection into Practice: Achieving and Sustaining Zero-Deficit Quality Goals*, pp.15–16. For the complete report or more information, visit The Advisory Board Company at www.advisory.com.

Agency for Healthcare Research and Quality. TeamSTEPPS®: Strategies and Tools to Enhance Performance and Patient Safety. Rockville, MD: Agency for Healthcare Research and Quality. http://www.ahrq.gov/qual/teamstepps/ Accessed on 1/11/2012.

Cardo, D., Dennehy, P.H., Halverson, P., *et al.* (2010) Moving toward elimination of healthcare-associated infections: a call to action. *Am. J. Infect. Control 38*:671–5.

Centers for Medicare and Medicaid Services. *Hospital Inpatient Quality Reporting Program.* CMS Website http://www.cms.gov/HospitalQualityInits/08_Hospital-RHQDAPU.asp

Department of Health and Human Services. Partnership for Patients. http://www.healthcare.gov/news/factsheets/2011/04/partnership04122011a.html Accessed on 1/15/2012

Division of Healthcare Quality Promotion; National Center for Emerging, Zoonotic, and Infectious Diseases; Centers for Disease Control and Prevention; Public Health Service; US Department of Health and Human Services. (2011) National Healthcare Safety Network (NHSN) Report, data summary for 2010, device-associated module, issued December 2011. *Am. J. Infect. Control 39*:798–816.

Fraser, V.J. (2002) Starting to learn about the costs of nosocomial infections in the new millenium: where do we go from here? *Infect. Control Hospital Epidemiol. 23*:174–6.

Gawande, A. (2007). *Better. A Surgeon's Notes on Performance.* New York: Picador.

Gurses, A.P., Xiao, Y., Seidl, K., *et al.* (2008) Systems ambiguity and guideline compliance: A qualitative study of how intensive care units follow evidence-based guidelines to reduce healthcare-associated infections. *Quality and Safety in Health Care 17*:351–9.

Hollenbeak, C.S., Murphy, D., Dunagan, W.C. and Fraser, V.J. (2002) Nonrandom selection and the attributable cost of surgical-site infections. *Infect. Control Hospital Epidemiol. 23*:177–182.

Institute of Medicine. (2000) *To Err Is Human: Building a Safer Health System.* Washington, DC: National Academies Press.

Klevens, R.M., Edwards, J.R., *et al.* (2007) Estimating health care-associated infections and deaths in U.S. hospitals, 2002. *Public Health Reports 122*:160–166.

Kohut, K. Guide for the prevention of mediastinitis surgical site infections following cardiac surgery: an elimination guide. Available from: http://www.apic.org/Content/NavigationMenu/PracticeGuidance/APICEliminationGuides/Mediastinitis_logo.pdf. Accessed January 9, 2012.

National Quality Forum (NQF). (2010) *Safe Practices for Better Healthcare—2010 Update: A Consensus Report.* Washington, DC: NQF.

Perencevich, E.N., Stone, P.W., Wright, S.B., *et al.* (2007) Raising standards while watching the bottom line: making a business case for infection control. *Infect. Control Hosp. Epidemiol. 28*:1121–1133.

Preas, M.A., Custer, M., Rew, C., Hebden, J.N., *et al.* (2011) Economic Impact of a Dedicated Nurse Champion in Reducing Catheter-Associated Bloodstream Infections. Presented at the National Conference of the Association of Professionals in Infection Control, June, 2011, Baltimore, Maryland.

Pronovost, P., Needham, D., Berenholtz, S., *et al.* (2006) An intervention to decrease catheter-related bloodstream infections in the ICU. *N. Eng. J. Med. 355*:2725–2732.

Rebmann, T. and Kohut, K. (2011) Preventing mediastinitis surgical site infections: executive summary of the Association for Professionals in Infection Control and Epidemiology's elimination guide. *Am. J. Infect. Control 39*:529–31.

Scheckler, W.E., Brimhall, D., Buck, A.S., *et al.* (1998) Requirements for infrastructure and essential activities of infection control and epidemiology in hospitals: a consensus panel report. *Am. J. Infect. Control 26*(1):47–60.

Scott, R.D. (2009) The Direct Medical Costs of Healthcare-Associated Infections in US Hospitals and the Benefits of Prevention. Division of Healthcare Quality Promotion; National Center for Preparedness, Detection, and Control of Infectious Diseases; Centers for Disease Control and Prevention, March 2009.

Streed, S.A. (2011) Metrics and management: two unresolved problems on the pathway to healthcare-associated infection elimination. *Am. J. Infect. Control 39*:678–84.

CHAPTER 2

Safe Infection Control in the Workplace

CAROL PATTON, PhD., RN, FNP and
DENISE M. KORNIEWICZ, Phd., RN, FAAN

The case study used for this chapter will explore the legal issues associated with safety and infection control. Topics include the National Institute of Occupational Safety & Health (NIOSH), employment guidelines, needle stick injuries, and personal responsibilities associated with safe patient practices.

2.1. CASE PRESENTATION

Kathy is a certified registered nurse anesthetist who has been working in the operating room for many years and provides intraoperative anesthesia during surgical procedures at a small, rural, hospital. Kathy is concerned about her safety and the safety of others in the operating room, as many nurses and other healthcare providers appear (in her opinion) to "take unnecessary chances and risks" when working with potentially harmful bloodborne pathogens common to healthcare settings. Kathy knows all hospital employees receive an annual update on infection control practices and safety. particularly when it comes to needle sticks and using personal protective equipment.

During the annual update, a variety of information is reiterated, updates are explained, and unit specific information is distributed. For example, operating room personnel must sign a form indicating they know how and understand when to use personal protective equipment, with particular focus on universal precaution techniques. Kathy knows that while some healthcare professionals do not see the need for the annual program, the updates and reminders are essential for preventing the spread of infectious diseases.

One of the main areas of emphasis during the annual update falls on reiterating the standards for healthcare workers developed in 1986 by the Occupational Safety and Health Administration (OSHA). Kathy knows that many of the OSHA standards were created to protect providers from pathogens to which they have a higher risk of being exposed because of their work, such as Hepatitis B, Hepatitis C, and HIV. Kathy believes the updates are necessary because she personally witnessed a nurse starting a preoperative peripheral intravenous access (IV) without using gloves. Kathy approached the nurse and called her aside to ask why she was risking exposure to blood and potentially disease. The nurse responded, "Because I just cannot start an IV with those bulky gloves". Kathy does not understand why this nurse will not use personal protective equipment to prevent exposure to potentially lethal infections.

2.2. ESSENTIAL CONTENT FOR SAFE INFECTION CONTROL IN THE WORKPLACE

According to The National Institute for Occupational Safety and Health (NIOSH), healthcare workers constitute over 18 million workers, of which 80% are female. Healthcare workplace hazards consist of numerous exposures to potential harms (CDC, 2012). NIOSH also notes that "cases of non-fatal occupational injury and illness among healthcare workers are among the highest of any industry sector" (NIOSH, 2012). The most common healthcare work place hazards that have legal implications include: needlestick and back injuries, latex allergies, violence and stress.

While many healthcare organizations have procedures and policies in place to protect healthcare workers from infectious disease through promoting safe infection control practices, there are few organizations that require healthcare workers to demonstrate mastery of safe infection control practice behaviors (Nielsen and Austin, 2005). It was not until 1985 that the first formally adopted Federal guidelines were developed to protect healthcare workers, identified as Standard Precautions (Tarrac, 2008). Standard Precautions became the fundamental foundation by which healthcare worker and patient safety programs were originated in an effort to increase protection from infectious disease. Standard Precautions serve as a guide for healthcare worker safety and protect patients from acquiring healthcare associated infections (HAIs) when properly implemented. Standard Precautions serve as a line of defense in controlling the spread of infection in healthcare settings. The development of Standard Precautions largely came about to protect healthcare workers, as well as patient populations, from becoming infected with HIV/AIDS. Over time, the title of Standard Precautions evolved into Universal Precautions because blood and body fluids from any patient can potentially be infectious.

Kathy is concerned about her safety and the safety of others in the operating room, as many nurses and other healthcare providers appear (in her opinion) to "take unnecessary chances and risks" when working with potentially harmful bloodborne pathogens common to healthcare settings.

Universal Precautions and initiatives to protect healthcare workers and patients from infectious disease are based on the Epidemiological Triad, often referred to as the EPI Triad. The Epidemiological Triad examines the relationship between host, agent, and environment (Fos, 2011). In order to interrupt the cycle of infection, there must be a change or alteration in one of the three components of the EPI triad. To create a culture of healthcare worker and patient safety with respect to infectious disease, information from research studies can be incorporated into healthcare system policies to foster a culture of safety. For example, educating healthcare workers about effective infection prevention strategies will provide them with the knowledge and methods needed to protect themselves and patients from pathogens in the healthcare setting. Educational initiatives must be meticulously cultivated and transparent to employees to create a culture of safety resulting in successful infection control. Healthcare workers must be held accountable for consistent implementation of behaviors that foster and promote a culture of safe infection control practice.

One of the major challenges in creating a culture that embraces safe infection control practices include initiatives that are more than just "risk management". "Risk management is a system for dealing with the likelihood that a future event will cause some kind of harm in the healthcare environment" (Flores, 2006). Unfortunately, there is a risk—to employees and patients—of acquiring infection in the healthcare setting; therefore, creating a culture that is "risk adverse" can result in safe infection control practices. Healthcare organizations currently track infection and other safety indicators to evaluate performance of patient outcomes. The additional performance standards associated with healthcare provider safety for infection control is required to create a culture of quality and safety.

2.3. EMPLOYER STANDARDS FOR BLOODBORNE PATHOGEN PRECAUTIONS

Kathy knows that many of the OSHA standards were created to protect providers from pathogens to which they have a higher risk of being exposed because of their work, such as Hepatitis B, Hepatitis C, and HIV. Kathy believes the updates are necessary because she personally witnessed a nurse starting a preoperative peripheral intravenous access (IV) without using gloves.

Prior to the development of Standard and Transmission-Based Precautions in the 1980s, there was confusion among employers as to what type of personal protective equipment (PPE) should be used in healthcare settings. For example, there was ambiguity among healthcare providers as to when to use gloves, type of glove, patient risk factors and for how long a glove should be used. Several issues related to the exposure of bloodborne pathogens—the rationale as to when, how or

TABLE 2.1. Key Components of Standard Precautions and Rationale for the Component.

Standard Precaution	Rationale for Standard Precautions
Treat every patient as potentially infectious and/or susceptible to infection.	Patient may have an infection present without visible signs or symptoms.
Handwashing prior to and after each patient encounter.	Handwashing remains the single-most important way to prevent the spread of microorganisms between and among healthcare workers and patients.
Wear gloves when in contact with any blood or body fluid, soiled or contaminated instruments or equipment, and when invasive procedures may occur.	Gloves protect the healthcare worker from infectious organisms that may be present in patient blood or body fluids.
Apply and use additional Personal Protective Equipment (PPE) to provide physical barriers when there is an index of even low suspicion that there may be exposure to blood and body fluid splashes.	Healthcare workers must wear proper PPE—including but not limited to goggles, face masks and/or aprons—to protect themselves in a preventive manner, knowing the types of patient or work encounters that expose them to blood and body fluid splashes.
Create a culture of safety for work practice when dealing with sharps, shards of glass or other potentially sharp objects.	Exposure risk is limited when equipment is properly handled.
Follow recommended organizational procedure/policy for handling and disposal of contaminated/dirty items.	Protect healthcare workers and patients from potential hazards from contaminated/dirty items.

why a healthcare provider would need to use PPE—was investigated. Table 2.1 provides the key concepts for standard precautions and the rationale.

2.4. PERSONAL PROTECTIVE EQUIPMENT (PPE)

It is readily apparent and well-documented in the research literature that there is no single best approach to creating safe infection control practice. However, proper use of Personal Protective Equipment (PPE) is essential for fostering effective infection control practices to promote healthcare worker and patient safety. The purpose of PPE in healthcare settings is to protect the worker from actual and potentially harmful agents by creating a barrier between the healthcare worker and the agent. There are five main types of PPE the healthcare workers must be prepared to use in order to protect themselves and others from infectious agents and other hazards (CDC, 2012). These include: gloves, gowns/aprons, masks, respirators and eyewear (Table 2.2). The CDC offers educational modules for PPE use in healthcare settings. The modules are designed to enable healthcare workers to select the proper PPE and to teach them how to safety apply and remove it.

Kathy approached the nurse and called her aside to ask why she was risking exposure to blood and potentially disease. The nurse responded "because I just cannot start an IV with those bulky gloves". Kathy does not understand why this nurse will not use personal protective equipment to prevent exposure to potentially lethal infections.

Ideally, ongoing assessment of proper application and use of the PPE, as well as follow-up surveillance, has been suggested in workplace environments. Consistent use of PPE provides additional safety for healthcare providers. However, the lack of consistent methods to monitor the use of PPE in healthcare settings has caused concern among healthcare administrators.

2.4.1. Latex Allergies: Patient or Healthcare Provider

Many of the safety protocols in healthcare organizations require the use of gloves for barrier protection. However, healthcare workers and patients may have an allergy to latex, which has traditionally been the

TABLE 2.2. PPE Mandated by OSHA and Considerations for Healthcare Workers.

Type of PPE Mandated by OSHA	Role in Providing Barrier Protection	Considerations
Gloves	Provide barriers to protect the hands	• There are different types of gloves for different purposes • Sterile or non-sterile • Determine if need to use single or double gloves • Choose vinyl, latex, nitrile or other, depending on work to be done and personal factors (Latex allergy) • Do not touch face or mask with contaminated gloves • Change gloves if they become torn or heavily soiled and always before starting the next task, even with the same patient • Discard gloves in the nearest appropriate receptacle and wash hands
Gowns/Aprons	Protect skin or clothing	• Don prior to patient contact, generally before entering the patient room • Be cautious not to spread contamination • Carefully remove and discard either at the doorway or just outside the patient room • Discard in a receptacle appropriate for the PPE • Immediately wash hands after removing the gown or apron • Gowns are made from different materials, so selection needs to be based on procedure and need (For example, isolation gowns are not fluid-impervious) • Sterile gown must be selected for sterile procedure or an invasive procedure • Must wear a fluid-resistant gown if arms can be exposed to blood or body fluids

(continued)

TABLE 2.2 (continued). PPE Mandated by OSHA and Considerations for Healthcare Workers.

Type of PPE Mandated by OSHA	Role in Providing Barrier Protection	Considerations
Masks	Protect the mouth and nose	• Selection is determined by the nature of the contact • Need to fully cover the nose and mouth and prevent fluid penetration • Must fit snugly over the nose and mouth • Preferably use mask with strong ties or adjustable elastic for secure fit and also flexible nose piece
Respirators	Protect the respiratory tract from airborne infectious agents	• Used when there is a need to filter the air before inhaling (Example, when exposed to a patient with known or suspected Mycobacterium tuberculosis) • Most commonly used respirators are N95, N99, or N100 particulate respirators • These devices have sub-micron filters that exclude particles smaller then 5 microns from entering the respiratory tract • Must consider the nature of the risk and exposure
Eyewear/Goggles	Protect eyes	• Goggles provide barrier protection • Do not rely on personal prescriptive eyewear for absolute protection(Example: Do not use your eye glasses as protection) • Should fit snugly over and around the eyes • Preferable to have anti-fog features for vision clarity and safety during procedures
Face Shields	Protect the face, mouth, nose, and eyes	• Typically used when added protection from splashes (For example, when irrigating a wound or suctioning secretions) is needed • Should cover the forehead, extend below the chin, and wrap around the side of the face

most commonly-used type of glove in the healthcare setting. The most compelling reason for awareness of latex allergies in healthcare workers and patient populations is because the immediate reaction is an IgE-mediated response that may result in anaphylaxis or death (Smith, Wallace, and Smith-Campbell, 2010).

2.4.2. Disposal and Handling of Soiled Equipment and Used Supplies

Major consideration for handling and discarding soiled and/or contaminated equipment and supplies are necessary for successful infection control in healthcare settings. Organizational policies and procedures should be consistent with federal guidelines. It should be known who made them, where they are available, and should be followed to ensure patient and healthcare worker safety. For example, information

TABLE 2.3. Major Resources for Assisting in Proper and Safe Handling and Disposal of Soiled Medical Equipment and Used Supplies.

National Center for Patient Safety, http://www.patientsafety.gov/patients.html
Safe Care Campaign, http://www.patientsafety.gov/ncpsexit.asp?url=www.safecare-campaign.org/SCC_2010/patients_01.html
Infection: Don't Pass It On, http://www.publichealth.va.gov/infectiondontpassiton/
Apply and use additional Personal Protective Equipment (PPE) to provide physical barriers when there is an index of even low suspicion that there may be exposure to blood and body fluid splashes.
Institute for Healthcare Improvement CDC Guide to How-to Guide: Improving Hand Hygiene, A Guide for Improving Practices among Health Care Workers, http://www.shea-online.org/Assets/files/IHI_Hand_Hygiene.pdf
Joint Commission Hazardous Materials and Waste Standards, http://www.health-leadersmedia.com/content/HOM-73264/Joint-Commission-Hazardous-Materials-and-Waste-Standards.html
National Patient Safety Foundation, http://www.npsf.org/updates-news-press/reducing-surgical-site-infections/
OSHA Occupation Exposure to Bloodborne Pathogens, http://www.osha.gov/pls/oshaweb/owadisp.show_document?p_id=811&p_table=PREAMBLES
Agency for Healthcare Research and Quality, http://www.hhs.gov/ash/initiatives/hai/incentives.html
Acello, B. The OSHA Handbook: Guidelines for Compliance in Health Care Facilities and Interpretive Guidelines for the Bloodborne Pathogens Standards (3rd ed.) Independence, KY: Cengage Learning.
American Society for Healthcare Risk Management, http://www.nap.edu/openbook.php?isbn=0309039754

for specific cleansing agents required for various exposures should be readily available in areas where exposures may occur to prevent health-care worker harm. Additionally, numerous federal and state resources are available for healthcare organizations to ensure their policies meet established safety criteria. Table 2.3 highlights some of the major resources for assisting in proper and safe handling and disposal of soiled medical equipment and used supplies.

Healthcare worker safety may also be jeopardized by exposure to chemicals used to clean or disinfect soiled medical equipment. For example, a major metropolitan hospital experienced an increased incidence and prevalence of asthma in nurses and technicians using gluteraldehyde to sterilize instruments used in the G.I. lab. The issue occurred as a result of inadequate ventilation in the sterilization room where the G.I. instruments were cleaned and sterilized. In this specific example, there were clinical issues and challenges associated with healthcare worker safety.

2.5. SHARPS INJURIES

Sharps injuries to healthcare workers are caused by needle sticks or other sharp instruments puncturing the skin while providing care. These types of injuries continue to occur frequently and remain a major risk for transmission of bloodborne pathogens despite several initiatives to decrease and minimize such injuries (Muralidhard *et al.*, 2010). For example, from 1984 to 1996 there were in excess of 1,000 patents issued for safety devices designed to prevent percutaneous needle sticks, but in 2012 there continues to be risks associated with handling sharp medical equipment (Brown, 2005, p. 22). Furthermore, the CDC explicitly outlines a method to prevent sharps injuries in their *Workbook for Designing, Implementing and Evaluating a Sharps Injury Prevention Program* that identifies major issues in a sharps injury prevention program and provides a Toolkit for healthcare organizations to develop a comprehensive sharps injury prevention program (Centers for Disease Control, 2008). Table 2.4 highlights major causes of percutaneous injuries to healthcare workers.

Despite major advancements in safety features of equipment like "needleless systems" and enhancements in medical supply technology for nearly two decades, there is still no substitute for improving education and creating a culture of safety and quality in all healthcare delivery systems (Brown, 2005).

TABLE 2.4. *Major Causes of Percutaneous Injuries to Healthcare Workers (Muralidhard et al., 2010).*

- Type and design of needles used for blood collection
- Intravenous cannulas
- Intravenous connection devices
- Recapping activity
- Handling and transferring specimens
- Collisions between healthcare workers with sharps during event clean-up
- Passing or handing off devices
- Failure to properly dispose of sharps in proper receptacles

2.5.1. Healthcare Worker Values and Beliefs on Reporting Sharps Injuries

Sharp objects in the healthcare setting injure approximately 600,000 to 800,000 healthcare workers annually, potentially exposing them to life threatening bloodborne pathogens (Anderson, 2010). Another staggering statistic is that more than half of all reported sharps injuries in healthcare workers go unreported. Strategies to engage healthcare workers in reporting sharps injuries require an investment in education and a culture of continuous awareness to protect injured healthcare workers' health. The first reported and verified case of HIV being contracted by a healthcare worker via a needle stick injury occurred in 1984 (Anderson, 2010). Due to the risks encountered by healthcare workers related to sharps injuries, OSHA began developing standards and protocols to prevent exposure to bloodborne pathogens, Congress passed the Needle Stick Safety and Prevention Act, and also some states began to integrate healthcare worker safety mandates into labor codes (Anderson, 2010). Safety-engineered devices have made substantive impacts in preventing sharps injuries. However, more than safety-engineered technology and devices are needed to reach sustainable levels of healthcare worker safety related to sharps injuries (Tuma and Sepkowitz, 2006).

2.6. DESIGNING PROGRAMS OF HEALTHCARE WORKER SAFETY

The causes of a majority of healthcare worker injuries are multifactorial and complex with no simple solution. According to Schulte *et al.* (2012), the complexity between the interaction of occupational and personal risk factors is frequently underutilized when developing workplace safety interventions. It is essential when designing, implementing, and evaluating healthcare worker safety programs that there is assessment and integration of both occupational risk factors (ORF) and personal risk factors (PRF). This approach is critical for the well-being and safety of healthcare worker and patients, and for maintaining a robust national healthcare workforce (Schulte *et al.*, 2012).

2.6.1. Elements of Models for Success in Safe Infection Control Practices

Regardless of all that is known regarding safe infection control practices, still healthcare workers may not fully embrace the infection control procedures and policies at the federal or organizational level. Clearly, the majority of healthcare organizations provide annual—if not more frequent—healthcare worker mandatory universal precaution education programs. Additionally, the Centers for Disease Control (CDC) continuously performs research to improve healthcare worker and patient safety. However, legal issues and challenges lie in fostering and promoting adherence to the standards to reduce the transmission of infectious diseases in healthcare settings.

2.7. SURVEILLANCE AND BEHAVIORAL-BASED PERFORMANCE OF HEALTHCARE WORKERS

Key elements involved in supporting healthcare worker adherence to a culture of safety include, but are not limited to, administrative and leadership support at all levels of the healthcare organization (McLaughlin, Johnson and Sollecito, 2012). Leadership in the organization must make a commitment to providing necessary and essential equipment for healthcare worker safety, monitoring healthcare worker adherence to policies, and management support to create and sustain a culture of infection control safety (Beam *et al.*, 2011; Casanova *et al.*, 2011; Nichol *et al.*, 2012; Weiner-Well *et al.*, 2011). Infection control and prevention is a role for which each healthcare worker needs to be educated and held accountable. Quality control in infectious disease must be ongoing and a continuous quality improvement initiative is an inherent component of the organizational culture and professional behavior from every healthcare worker all the time. Table 2.5 indicates key components of a comprehensive infection control continuous quality improvement initiative to facilitate creation and maintenance of replicable and sustainable healthcare worker behavior change.

TABLE 2.5. Key Components of a Comprehensive Infection Control Continuous Quality Improvement Initiative.

- Commitment from senior healthcare administrators at the Macro level to organizational support for comprehensive infection control continuous quality improvement initiative
- Select champions from the Micro system level to drive the evidence-based infection control culture and change
- Provision of human and financial resources to support the comprehensive infection control continuous quality improvement initiative in the annual budget
- Provide human and financial resources to support attendance at local, regional, national and international meetings to advance infection control processes and education for sustainable healthcare worker behavior change
- Make certain project goals are linked to the organizational mission and philosophy and are developed collaboratively with key stakeholders and consensus is reached
- Make certain project goals are behaviorally measurable, time specific, and outcomes are clear to all
- Perform tests of change and monitor through ongoing surveillance to determine adherence of all healthcare workers
- Link healthcare worker performance to annual performance appraisal
- Be transparent in the process and share aggregate data with all healthcare workers
- Provide outcome data monthly to all healthcare workers
- Evaluate the impact of change with measurement instruments that are valid and reliable

2.8. CREATING A CULTURE OF SAFE INFECTION CONTROL PRACTICES

Safe infection control practices do not happen without careful thought and purposive design in any healthcare organization. There must be a commitment to quality and safety to purposefully and deliberately plan, design, implement, and evaluate the culture of safe infection control practices (Berryman, 2006; Duval, 2010; Chalmers and Straub, 2006; Wiseman, 2006). Every healthcare professional has a code of ethics that they embrace upon completion of their professional education or training. While these may differ slightly from profession to profession, there are commonalities.

2.8.1. Legal Issues with Safety and Infection Control Practices

There are federal regulatory guidelines and organizational proce-dures/policies in place to protect healthcare workers and patient populations and yet—as the case study demonstrates—there remain healthcare workers who do not practice based on the safety and infection control guidelines. While intellectually a healthcare worker may know the proper evidence-based procedures/policies to follow with respect to safe infection control practices for self and others, it remains a mystery why more healthcare workers do not embrace and commit to behavioral actions that apply these procedures and policies.

2.9. REFERENCES

Amarasekera, M., Rathnamalala, N., Samaraweera, S. and Jinadasa, M. (2010). Prevalence of latex allergy among healthcare workers. *International Journal of Occupational Medicine and Environmental Health, 23*(4):391–396.

Anderson, J.M. (2010). Needle stick injuries: Prevention and education key. *Journal of Controversial Medical Claims, 15*(3):12–19.

Beam, E.L., Gibbs, S.G., Boulter, K.C., Beckerdite, M.E. and Smith, P.W. (2011). A method for evaluating health care worker's personal protective equipment technique. *American Journal of Infection Control 39*(5):415–420.

Berryman, F. (2006). Infection control principles. *Nursing Standard 20*:66.

Brown, M. (2005). Optimize I.V. infusion safety with a comprehensive approach. *IT Solutions,* October 2005, pp. 19–22.

Casanova, L.M., Rutala, W.A., Weber, D.J. and Sobsey, M.D. (2011). Effect of single-versus double-gloving on virus transfer to health care workers' skin and clothing during removal of personal protective equipment. *American Journal of Infection Control 40*:369–374.

Centers for Disease Control. (2008). A workbook for designing, implementing, and evaluating a sharps injury prevention program. http://www.cdc.gov/sharpssafety/pdf/sharpsworkbook_2008.pdf

Chalmers, C. and Straub, M. (2006). Standard principles for preventing and controlling infection. *Nursing Standard, 20*(23):57–66.

Cohen, N.L. and Patton, C.M. (2006). Worker safety and gluteraldehyde in the gastrointestinal lab environment. *Gastroenterol Nurs., 29*(2):100–4.

Duval, L. (2010). Infection control 101. *Nephrology Nursing Journal, 37*(5): 485–489.

Fos, P.J. (2011). *Health and disease. In Epidemiology foundations: The science of public health,* pp. 35–51. San Francisco, CA: Jossey-Bass.

Healthcare workers. (2012). CDC Web Site. Retrieved from http://www.cdc.gov/niosh/topics/healthcare/

Loeppke, R. (2008). The value of health and the power of prevention. *International Journal Workplace Health Management, 12*:95–108.

McLaughlin, C.P., Johnson, J.K. and Sollecito, W.A. (2012). *Implementing continuous quality improvement in healthcare: A global casebook.* Sudbury, MA: Jones & Bartlett.

Muralidhard, S., Singh, P.K., Jain, R.K., Malhotra, M. and Bala, M. (2010). Needle stick injuries among health care workers in a tertiary care hospital of India. *Indian J. Med. Res., 131*:405–410.

Nichol, K., McGeer, A., Bigelow, P., O'Brien-Palles, L. and Holness, D.L. (2012).

Behind the mask: Determinants of nurses' adherence to facial protective equipment. *American Journal of Infection Control 41*:(1):8-13.

Nielsen, D. and Austin, J. (2005). Behavior-based safety: Improvement opportunities in hospital safety. *Professional Safety*, pp. 33–37.

Niggemann, B. (2010). IgE-mediated latex allergy- An exciting and instructive piece of allergy history. *Pediatric Allergy and Immunology, 21*:997–1001.

Pavkovic, S., Goetz, K., Prachand, A. and Stanley, S. (2011). Improving risk manager performance and promoting patient safety with high-reliability principles. In: *Priniciples of Risk Management and Patient Safety*, pp. 343–349. B.J. Youngberg (Ed.). Sudbury, MA: Jones & Bartlett.

Schulte, P.A., Pandalai, S., Wulsin, V. and Chun, H. (2012). Interaction of occupational and personal risk factors in workforce health and safety. *American Journal of Public Health, 102*:434–448.

Smith, K., Wallace, A. and Smith-Campbell, B. (2010). What you should know about latex allergy. *The Nurse Practitioner, 29*:24.

Stankovic, A. (2011). Protection against needlestick injuries: Active or passive safety? *Medical Laboratory Observer, 43*(9):40, 51.

Tabak, N., Shiaabana, A.M. and Shasha, S. (2006). The health beliefs of hospital staff and the reporting of needlestick injury. *Issues in Clinical Nursing, 15*:1228–1239.

Tuma, S. and Sepkowitz, K.A. (2006). Efficacy of safety-engineered device implementation in the prevention of percutaneous injuries: A review of published studies. *Healthcare Epidemiology, 42*:1159–1170.

Upshaw, V.M., Kaluzny, A.D. and McLaughlin, C.P. (2006). CQI, transformation, and the "Learning Organization". In: *Continuous Quality Improvement in Healthcare* (3rd ed.), pp. 191–210. C.P. McLaughin and A.D. Kaluzny (Eds.). Sudbury, MA: Jones & Bartlett.

Weiner-Well, Y., Galuty, M., Rudensky, B., Schlesinger, Y., Attias, D. and Yinnon, A.M. (2011). Nursing and physician attire as possible source of nosocomial infections. *American Journal of Infection Control, 39*:555–559.

Wiseman, S. (2006). Prevention and control of healthcare-associated infection. *Nursing Standard, 20*(38):41–45.

Youngberg, B. (2011). *Creating a Mindfulness of Patient Safety among Physicians Through Education*, pp. 375–395. Sudbury, MA: Jones & Bartlett.

CHAPTER 3

Patient Safety and the Chain of Infection

JOAN HEBDEN RN, MS, CIC

This chapter will include a case study that highlights the infectious disease process, indirect and direct transmission of microorganisms and the facts associated with infection and communicable diseases.

3.1. CASE PRESENTATION

Joan is a nurse practitioner in the Neonatal Intensive Care Unit (NICU) of a major academic medical center and is serving as the unit's admission officer for the day. She receives a call from the neonatal transport team that a local community hospital is in need of two beds for twins that were delivered emergently to a 19 year old with HELLP (hemolysis, elevated liver enzymes, low platelet count) syndrome at 26 weeks gestation. The birth weight for Twin A is 860 grams and for Twin B is 790 grams and both infants are requiring mechanical ventilation. Maternal history is positive for incarceration for the first three months of the pregnancy and a history of intravenous drug use with a negative screen for human immunodeficiency virus. A toxicology screen at the local hospital was negative.

The NICU is a 40-bed unit with 30 beds for intensive care and 10 beds for step-down care. The 30 bed unit is comprised of four pods, each with 7 bed spaces, and 2 single bed isolation rooms. Each of the pods is designated to provide care to infants with specific clinical needs: extremely low birthweight ELBW (< 1000 gram), very low birth weight VLBW (1001–1500 gram), surgical and general care. Currently, the ICU has a census of 28 infants and the bed spaces are full in the ELBW pod. The two available bed spaces are in the general and surgical pods. Joan and the charge nurse confer on the physical placement and management of the twins. Both are cognizant of the complex medical care that these premature infants will require for several months and want spatial proximity to support family visitation and bonding. Joan is concerned that the history of incarceration may have placed the mother at risk for colonization with methicillin-resistant *S. aureus* (MRSA) with possible acquisition by the twins. Therefore, she wants Contact Isolation precautions initiated until admission screening for MRSA can be performed. The birth weight of the twins and the need for mechanical ventilation and umbilical artery and vein catheterization warrants their placement in the ELBW pod. An assessment of the occupants of the ELBW pod is completed and a decision is made to transfer two infants that have recently been weaned from the ventilator to the other ICU bed spaces. The charge nurse points out that with the remaining five infants and the new admissions all on ventilators, as well as the order for Contact Isolation precautions for the twins, the pod will be crowded.

As the twins are en route to the hospital, the charge nurse quickly mobilizes resources to move the infants and to clean the vacated bed spaces in the ELBW pod. While the cleaning is being completed, the twins arrive and Joan is called to begin the admission process. Joan informs the admitting nurse that Contact Isolation precaution signs, gowns and gloves are needed at the bedsides of the twins. However, due to the critical condition of the infants, the attending neonatologist and fellow have proceeded to provide care without protective attire. When Joan arrives at the bedsides of the twins, she notes that the alcohol hand sanitizer is not available and asks the charge nurse to obtain the product. After Joan performs hand hygiene and dons a gown and gloves, she proceeds to assist in the care of the most critically ill twin. She explains to the rest of the team that the twins may be colonized with MRSA and asks that they perform hand hygiene and observe Contact Precautions. The admission process proceeds and the twins are stabilized. At this point, the mother is allowed to see the infants. Joan and the admitting nurse explain the importance of hand hygiene before and after contact with each twin and the rationale for Contact Isolation precautions. Joan asks the mother if she has ever been told she has MRSA or been tested for the organism. The mother states that she had a nasal swab performed at the transferring hospital but was not told the result. Joan makes a note in the twin's care plan to follow-up on this result and to ensure that admission nasal screening was performed on the twins.

In preparation for the change of shift, Joan and the charge nurse round in the unit. The charge nurse expresses concern about the crowdedness of the ELBW pod and states that staffing for the next shift is short due to a sick call-in. Joan recommends that the ELBW pod be provided with a minimum of four nurses to ensure that isolation precautions are maintained. When Joan arrives on the unit the next morning, she is notified that one of the infants who were transferred from the ELBW pod on the previous day has a positive sputum culture for multi-drug resistant *Acinetobacter baumannii*. Although this infant is now extubated and appears well, Joan is concerned about the less than optimal cleaning that occurred in the pod before the twins were admitted. She requests an additional cleaning of the room by Environmental Services.

3.2. ESSENTIAL CONTENT FOR INFECTION CONTROL SKILLS

Preventable healthcare associated infections (HAIs) occur with an alarming frequency in US hospitals, affecting an estimated 5–10% of hospitalized patients (Klevens, 2007). The risk of acquiring an HAI is particularly high for patients who need prolonged and complex medical care. Hospital-level factors that contribute to HAI risk include exposure to environmental flora, particularly antibiotic-resistant bacteria, through contaminated hands of healthcare providers or inanimate surfaces or equipment, nurse staffing, overcrowding, and the use of invasive medical devices. Individual factors that contribute to HAI risk include age, immune status, antibiotic use, and severity of illness (Figure 3.1).

This chapter will address the inter-related elements needed for transmission of infection within a healthcare setting: a source of infectious microorganisms, a susceptible host with a portal of entry receptive to the infecting agent, and a mode of transmission for the agent (Siegel, 2007). Infection prevention measures to break "the chain of infection" by altering the host, the environment or the agent will be emphasized.

3.2.1. The Host

Joan is concerned that the history of incarceration may have placed the mother at risk for colonization with methicillin-resistant *S. Aureus* (MRSA) with possible acquisition by the twins that were delivered emergently at 26 weeks gestation. The birth weight for Twin A is 860 grams and for Twin B is 790 grams and both infants are requiring mechanical ventilation.

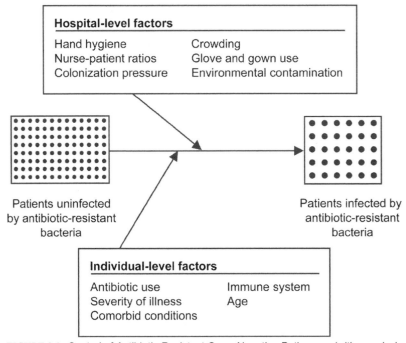

FIGURE 3.1. *Control of Antibiotic Resistant Gram-Negative Pathogens (with permission from Lautenbach, Practical Healthcare Epidemiology, Chapter 18, Harris A, Thom K, University of Chicago Press).*

Extremely low birth weight neonates represent a particularly vulnerable patient population who are at risk for HAIs. As with other critically ill patient populations, physiologic instability, the use of invasive devices for medical management and exposure to broad spectrum antibiotics contribute to the risk of infectious complications. Patient factors that increase the risk of infection include extremes of age, diabetes, poor nutritional status, malignant disorders, and immune deficiencies (Siegel, 2007). The intrinsic risk factor of immunosuppression is enhanced in the neonate who is deprived of many of the maternally acquired immunoglobulin G antibodies (Brady, 2005). The use of medications that alter normal flora, such as corticosteroids, gastric acid suppressors and antibiotics also increase susceptibility to infection. Impairment of the skin due to developmental immaturity or integrity disruption from surgery or the use of invasive devices alters a primary host defense against infection. Advances in treatment have increased survival of critically ill patients, leading to prolonged exposure and colonization with exogenous microorganisms from the hands of healthcare workers and hospital flora. Progression of colonization to infection varies from patient to patient and is dependent on the patients' immune status at the time of exposure to the infectious agent, interaction between pathogens and virulence factors intrinsic to the agent.

3.2.2. Sources of Infecting Agents

The birth weight of the twins and the need for mechanical ventilation and umbilical artery and vein catheterization warrants their placement in the ELBW pod . . .

Hospitalized patients can be exposed to pathogenic bacteria, viruses or fungi from a variety of sources. Human reservoirs include patients, healthcare workers, household members and other visitors. The source individuals may have an active infection, be transiently or chronically colonized or may be in the incubation period of an infectious disease. Other reservoirs include endogenous flora residing on the patients' skin, mucous membranes, gastrointestinal tract or respiratory tract. Inanimate environmental sources, such as patient room surfaces and equipment that have become contaminated, also are implicated in the transmission of infecting agents. An additional source of infection that is unique to neonates is the vertical transmission of microorganisms, such as Group B Streptococcus or Herpes simplex virus, from mother to infant derived from the birth canal.

3.2.3. Means of Transmission

Joan informs the admitting nurse that Contact Isolation precaution signs, gowns and gloves are needed at the bedsides of the twins. However, due to the critical condition of the infants, the attending neonatologist and fellow have proceeded to provide care without protective attire. When Joan arrives at the bedsides of the twins, she notes that the alcohol hand sanitizer is not available and asks the charge nurse to obtain the product.

There are three principal routes of transmission associated with the spread of infection in the healthcare setting which vary by type of organism. Contact transmission is the most frequent mode of transmission and is divided into two subgroups: direct and indirect contact. Direct contact involves a direct body surface-to-body surface contact and physical transfer of microorganisms between a susceptible host and an infected or colonized person, such as occurs in the performance of direct patient care activities, such as bathing a patient. Indirect contact involves transfer of an infectious agent through a contaminated intermediate object such as patient care equipment, toys or instruments, or the hands of healthcare professionals (HCPs). Recent literature suggests that healthcare professionals' clothing, including lab coats and isolation gowns, become contaminated with multi-drug resistant bacteria (e.g., MRSA, VRE, and *Acinetobacter baumannii*) and may contribute to the transmission of these organisms (Harris and Thom, 2010). Droplet transmission is a form of contact transmission, as some infectious agents that are spread by large droplets are also transmitted by direct and indirect contact routes. An example of a droplet transmitted disease, influenza, can be transmitted by respiratory droplets that are generated when an infected person coughs, sneezes or talks or during the performance of a procedure such as suctioning or intubation. The droplets are propelled a short distance, generally defined as 3 feet, and can be deposited directly onto the mucous membranes of a susceptible host. Additionally, the infectious droplets settle onto environmental surfaces, which can then be touched by individuals who self-inoculate their mucous membranes. Airborne transmission is associated with the dispersal of small droplets or droplet nuclei over long distances by air currents which may be inhaled by a susceptible host. The prevention of airborne diseases, such as tuberculosis, requires special air handling and ventilation systems and the use of respirators by HCPs.

3.2.4. Factors Enhancing Transmission

3.2.4.1. Nurse Staffing

> The charge nurse expresses concern about the crowdedness of the ELBW pod and states that staffing for the next shift is short due to a sick call-in. Joan recommends that the ELBW pod be provided with a minimum of four nurses to ensure that isolation precautions are maintained.

Numerous studies have illustrated an association between higher rates of HAIs and low nurse staffing levels. Fridkin *et al.* (1996) identified an increased patient-to-nurse ratio as an independent risk factor for central line-associated bloodstream infections among surgical intensive care unit patients. A case-control study conducted to investigate a 6-week outbreak of *Enterobacter cloacae* in a 15-bed NICU identified overcrowding and understaffing to be associated with the infections

(Harbarth, 1999). This study highlighted a decrease in hand washing compliance during periods of high workload demands. The findings from these papers and other research documenting that problems with nurse staffing are associated with adverse patient outcomes, including HAIs, led to a working group meeting on the issue convened by the Division of Healthcare Quality Promotion, Centers for Disease Control and Prevention. Additionally, a Category 1B recommendation for appropriate nurse staffing in the intensive care units has been included in the 2011 CDC Guidelines for the Prevention of Intravascular Catheter-Related Infections. The evidence is compelling that adequate bedside nursing staff influences the quality of patient care (Jackson, 2002). In respect to HAI prevention and control, adequate staff makes it more likely that hand hygiene, use of standard and transmission-based precautions and use of best practices will be adhered to correctly and consistently.

3.2.4.2. Overcrowding

The NICU is a 40-bed unit with 30 beds for intensive care and 10 beds for step-down care. The 30 bed unit comprises four pods, each with 7 bed spaces, and 2 single bed isolation rooms. Each of the pods is designated to provide care to infants with specific clinical needs: extremely low birth weight ELBW (< 1000 gram), very low birth weight VLBW (1001–1500 gram), surgical and general care. Currently, the ICU has a census of 28 infants and the bed spaces are full in the ELBW pod. The two available bed spaces are in the general and surgical pods. Joan and the charge nurse confer on the physical placement and management of the twins.

Overcrowding in multi-bed rooms, such as in a NICU, may occur as a result of unexpected admissions or emergent high-risk maternal transfers. The need for equipment such as ventilators and extracorporeal membrane oxygenation and infusion pumps to manage the complex care needs of these infants may reduce the allocated amount of bed space and contribute to equipment sharing. The designated amount of clearance between infant care beds is a minimum of 8 feet (2010). An increase above expected census and low nurse staffing levels may lead to inadequate equipment cleaning. A recent paper by Havill and colleagues found that nursing staff were not disinfecting equipment adequately (2011). Failure to perform adequate equipment cleaning can lead to the contamination of HCPs' hands, which in the absence of hand hygiene can become the vector for cross-transmission of potentially pathogenic organisms to patients.

3.2.5. Compliance with Hand Hygiene and Standard Precautions

After Joan performs hand hygiene and dons a gown and gloves, she proceeds to assist in the care of the most critically ill twin.

Hand hygiene is recognized as the single most important practice to reduce the transmission of infectious agents with guidelines from both the Centers for Disease Control and the World Health Organization serving as compliance standards for The Joint Commission (TJC) National Patient Safety Goal (NPSG) 07.01.01 to reduce HAIs. Improvement in hand hygiene practice has been associated with the reduction of HAIs as well as decreases in the transmission of multi-drug resistant organisms. Although the use of an antimicrobial soap or alcohol-based hand rub is indicated before and after direct contact with patients, poor compliance with hand hygiene has been widely documented. For example, in the NICU setting, compliance has been reported to be less than 50% (Cohen, 2003). In order to better understand the reasons for poor hand hygiene compliance among HCPs, researchers have begun to explore possible behavioral determinants. A qualitative study of NICU physicians and nurses conducted by Pessoa-Silva and colleagues (2005) revealed that intention to comply with hand hygiene guidelines was significantly related to perceived control over the difficulty of performing hand hygiene and a positive perception of superiors' valuing compliance with hand hygiene. A more recent study using structured interview questions with physicians, nurses and medical students found that hand hygiene behavior appears to be motivated by self-protection and a desire to clean oneself after performing a task that is viewed as dirty and that lack of positive role models hinders compliance (Erasmus, 2009). The authors concluded that further education of the HCPs focusing on patient protection would have little effect on compliance. They suggested that more sustainable improvements in hand hygiene would be achieved by modifying the environment with increased visibility of sinks and alcohol-based hand rubs and through incentives directed at senior staff who serve as role models. The NPSG stipulates that organizations have a hand hygiene policy as well as compliance monitoring and the provision of feedback. Hand hygiene is an essential component of Standard Precautions. Standard Precautions are based on the principle that all moist body substances may contain potentially transmissible infectious agents and are intended to be used with all patients. The use of gowns, gloves, masks and eye protection are to be worn by HCPs in anticipation of contact with body substances through direct patient contact or through contact with contaminated equipment or surfaces.

3.2.6. Compliance with Transmission-Based Precautions

The admission process proceeds and the twins are stabilized. At this point, the mother is allowed to see the infants. Joan and the admitting nurse explain the importance of hand hygiene before and after contact with each twin and the rationale for Contact Isolation precautions.

When the use of standard precautions will not interrupt the transmission of the infectious agent, the use of transmission-based precautions is indicated. In the case study example, Contact Precautions were ordered for the twins until the potential acquisition of MRSA from the mother could be determined. These precautions include hand hygiene, the wearing of gowns and gloves for each contact with the infant or their environment, disinfection of reusable patient care equipment and heightened environmental cleaning. The recommended use of Contact Precautions for the prevention of multi-drug resistant organism (MDRO) transmission is a key control strategy cited in the CDC Guidelines for the Prevention of MDROs as well as the Society for Healthcare Epidemiologists of America guidelines (Muto, 2003). MRSA is considered one of two major MDRO pathogens (enterococcus resistant to vancomycin is the other) with distinct genotypes associated with healthcare-associated and community-associated strains (CA-MRSA). Recent data from the CDC noted that the prevalence of MRSA acquisition in US hospitals increased from 48% in 1997 to 65% in 2007 (Burton, 2009). The emergence of CA-MRSA strains, which are termed USA300 and USA400, are associated with skin and soft tissue infections and are being seen with increasing frequency within healthcare facilities. As the majority of carriers of MRSA are asymptomatically colonized and may be undetected, active surveillance screening has been recommended as a part of a multi-faceted program to control transmission of MDROs in facilities with high-risk patient populations. In response to an increasing number of MRSA outbreaks in NICUs, the Chicago Department of Public Health convened a working group to develop consensus guidelines for infant management (Gerber, 2006). These guidelines recommend the use of Contact Precautions when caring for patients known or suspected to be MRSA-positive.

Maternal history is positive for incarceration for the first three months of the pregnancy and a history of intravenous drug use with a negative screen for human immunodeficiency virus.

In the case study, the admitting NP recognizes that incarceration is a risk factor for MRSA and appropriately places the twins on Contact Precautions until admission surveillance cultures are obtained and results available. The skin-to-skin exposure of multiple gestation infants to each other and to their mother contributes to the risk of colonization and infection with pathogenic bacteria (Siegel, 2007). In a recent study conducted to determine the risk of MRSA acquisition as a result of exposure to MRSA colonized infants, the authors found that placing a MRSA-positive infant on Contact Precautions reduced the overall odds of another patient becoming colonized by 35% (Geva, 2011).

The use of gloves and gowns by HCPs is a requirement of Contact Precautions. The prevention of hand contamination with appropriate glove use and the use of gowns to avoid contamination of unprotected skin and HCPs' clothing reduces the likelihood of transmission of potentially pathogenic bacteria to patients during the provision of care. Protective barriers frequently become contaminated with multi-drug resistant organisms either through direct patient contact or through contact with the patient environment. Snyder and colleagues (2008) identified that the degree of contamination of both gloves and gowns of staff caring for patients with MRSA and/or VRE was increased if contact with the respiratory tract or indwelling devices occurred. An important finding of these authors was that 3% of the HCPs' hands were contaminated with MRSA after the removal of their gloves and gowns, which substantiates the need to perform hand hygiene after barriers are removed. Several authors have examined the contamination of gloves and gowns with multi-drug resistant organisms (MDROs) from environmental surfaces. In a recent study by Morgan *et al.* (2011), *Acinetobacter baumannii* was the MDRO that most frequently contaminated the gloves and gowns of HCPs and environmental contamination was the major determinant of transmission of MDROs to HCPs' gloves and gowns. The authors cite compliance with Contact Precautions and aggressive environmental cleaning as important measures to control MDRO transmission.

3.2.7. Equipment and Environmental Decontamination Procedures

The report of a positive sputum culture for *A. baumannii* in a neonate transferred from the ELBW room appropriately raised the concern of the nurse practitioner in the case study. Thom *et al.* (2011) report that the surrounding environment of patients with multi-drug resistant *A. baumannii*, even among patients with a remote history of the organism, is frequently contaminated. Supply carts, floors, infusion pumps and ventilator touch pads were most commonly contaminated. These surfaces are often touched by HCPs who will contaminate their hands and clothing or their protective barriers, if worn. This contamination may contribute to the transmission of this emerging pathogen, which can cause all types of healthcare-associated infections.

Environmental cleaning is a critical component of a healthcare facility's comprehensive infection prevention and control program (IPC) and cleaning protocols and the disinfectants used must be approved by the IPC Committee. Based on increased reports of environmental contamination with MDROs and the prolonged survivability of these organisms on surfaces, researchers have begun to focus on the thoroughness of cleaning of patient rooms. Carling and colleagues (2007) evaluated the discharge cleaning of ICU rooms by targeting frequently touched surfaces and found that only 57% of the surfaces were adequately cleaned, with low rates of cleaning (< 30%) for sites likely to be contaminated with nosocomial pathogens, such as doorknobs, toilet area handholds and bedpan cleaners. An evaluation of inpatient non-ICU units found that the rate of cleaning adequacy ranged from 38–96% with a higher rate of adequate cleaning of high-touch surfaces in contact isolation rooms versus non-isolation rooms (Rupp, 2010).

These findings emphasize the need for education of environmental service workers on cleaning protocols and the importance of their work in preventing transmission of potentially pathogenic bacteria. The findings have also led to enhanced quality control measures, such as the placement of fluorescent markers on high-touch surfaces, which allow for real-time feedback and the reinforcement of correct techniques.

Nursing staff are instrumental in ensuring that reusable patient care equipment that is not the responsibility of environmental services is adequately cleaned and disinfected. Some of this equipment, such as glucometers and vital sign machines, are generally the responsibility of nursing. However, the cleaning of equipment such as infusion pumps and ventilators may be ambiguous if not clearly delineated. Whenever possible, patient care equipment used for isolation patients should be single-patient use and disposed of at discharge.

3.2.8. Patient and Family Education

Patients, family members and visitors are important partners in the prevention of transmission of infections in healthcare settings. Incorporating the importance of hand hygiene, respiratory/cough etiquette, and Standard Precautions into patient information materials upon admission with additional information provided about care protocols (e.g., Transmisson-based Precautions) as required, will engage and empower them to ensure that infection prevention practices are followed.

3.2.9. Antimicrobial Use

With more than 70 percent of the bacteria that cause HAIs being resistant to at least one of the drugs most commonly used to treat these infections, clinicians with prescribing authority are being asked to use antibiotics judiciously (CDC, 2001). Elimination of broad-spectrum antibiotics as soon as culture results are known, particularly those that impact the endogenous flora of the gastrointestinal tract and skin, is a practical way to reduce the contribution of antibiotic use on the selection of multi-drug resistant bacteria. An inherent component of the Campaign to Prevent Antimicrobial Resistance (2002) is the wise use of antimicrobials, which includes not only limiting the use of inappropriate agents, but also selecting the appropriate antibiotic, dosage, and duration of therapy to achieve optimal treatment efficacy.

3.3. INTERPRETATION/APPLICATION OF INFECTION CONTROL DATA

Advanced practice nurses (APNs) have assumed an increasing role as care providers in complex healthcare settings. This role requires an expert knowledge base that allows for the planning and provision of skilled and competent care. The prevention of HAIs and transmission of organisms to other patients is an essential component of each and every patient's plan of care, accomplished through implementation of the fundamental practices of infection control. These practices include: (1) serving as the primary resource to identify patient risk factors for infection; (2) performing, monitoring and assuring compliance with evidence-based best practices to reduce HAIs; (3) addressing administrative variables, such as nurse-to-patient ratios; (4) antimicrobial stewardship; and (5) fostering collaborative relationships with and providing oversight to workers responsible for environmental decontamination.

3.4. PATIENT SAFETY AND HEALTH SYSTEM: INFECTION CONTROL PRACTICES

HAIs continue to be the most common complication of hospitalization and their prevention has become a major focus of the national patient safety movement. Recognizing that infection transmission risks are present in all hospital settings and that not all HAIs can be prevented, healthcare providers (HCPs) are challenged on a daily basis to "break the chain of infection". The patient variables of age, immune status and severity of illness which contribute to host susceptibility are not modifiable. However, prompt identification and appropriate treatment of infection by HCPs can mitigate the risk of patient-to-patient transmission of pathogenic bacteria. Furthermore, important adjunctive measures such as careful screening of patients for potential infectious organisms/diseases with initiation of isolation, if warranted, and using antimicrobials wisely to avoid the alteration of normal endogenous flora and the emergence of multi-drug resistant bacteria reduce transmission risk. The reduction of exogenous transmission of organisms can be achieved with recommended hand hygiene practices and the proper use of protective barriers. However, despite the knowledge of best practices and the high educational level of healthcare workers, compliance is suboptimal (Farr, 2000) suggesting that environmental, e.g., increasing the visibility of sinks and alcohol-based rubs, and behavioral, e.g., real-time peer feedback of non-compliance and leaders who serve as role models, interventions are necessary to sustain practice change.

During the past decade, contaminated equipment and environmental surfaces have been cited as contributors to the transmission of multi-drug resistant organisms with enhanced cleaning included as a major infection control measure in halting outbreaks. This knowledge has helped to demonstrate to HCPs how contamination of their hands and gloves may occur, regardless of whether direct patient care was provided. Proper cleaning of the patient environment has become a campaign, "Clean Spaces, Healthy Patients", which is a collaborative between the Association for Professionals in Infection Control and the Association for the Healthcare Environment (AHE). The campaign is targeted to all healthcare personnel in any healthcare setting where the environment can be a source of disease transmission. This project is an example of infection preventionists and environmental services personnel working together to improve patient outcomes.

The engagement and empowerment of all healthcare staff is necessary to drive best practices for HAI prevention to the bedside of each and every patient. Through the skilled leadership of clinicians, such as APNs, who endorse these practices and serve as role models, the elimination of HAIs can become a reality.

3.5. SUMMARY POINTS

• Hand hygiene is the single most important procedure to prevent the spread of infection.
• Transmission of infection within a healthcare setting requires three elements: a source of an infecting agent, a susceptible host, and a mode of transmission for the agent.
• Sources of infecting agents include human reservoirs, inanimate environmental surfaces and patient care equipment.
• Factors enhancing transmission include low nurse-patient ratios, overcrowding, lack of compliance with hand hygiene and use of barrier precautions, antimicrobial use, and insufficient equipment and environmental surface cleaning.
• Achieving compliance with best practices to prevent HAIs requires an organizational culture focused on patient safety; sustaining compliance requires attention to the environmental and behavioral factors contributing to non-compliance.

3.6. REFERENCES

Brady, M.T. (2005) Health care-associated infections in the neonatal intensive care unit. *Am. J. Infect. Control 33*:268–75.

Burton, D.C., Edwards, J.R., Horan, T.C., *et al.* (2009) Methicillin-resistant Staphylococcus aureus central line-associated bloodstream infections in US intensive care units, 1997–2007. JAMA 301:727–736.

Carling, P.C., Parry, M.F. and Von Beheren, S.M., and Healthcare Environmental Hygiene Study Group. (2008) Identifying opportunities to enhance environmental cleaning in 23 acute care hospitals. *Infect Control Hosp Epidemiol 29*(1):1–7.

Centers for Disease Control and Prevention. (2001) Campaign to prevent antimicrobial resistance in healthcare settings: why a campaign? Atlanta, GA. Available at http://www.cdc.gov/drugresistance/healthcare/problem.htm. Accessed February 2012.

Cohen, B., Saiman, L., Cimiotti, J., *et al.* (2003) Factors associated with hand hygiene practices in two neonatal intensive care units. *Pediatr. Infect. Dis. J. 22*:494–499.

Erasmus, V., Brouwer, W., van Beeck, E.F., *et al.* (2009) A qualitative exploration of reasons for poor hand hygiene among hospital workers: lack of positive role models and of convincing evidence that hand hygiene prevents cross-infection. *Infect. Control Hosp. Epidemiol. 30*:415–19.

Farr, B.M. (2000) Reasons for noncompliance with infection control guidelines. *Infect. Control Hosp. Epidemiol. 21*(6):411–16.

Fridkin, S.K., Pear, S.M., Williamson, T.H., Galgianai, J.N. and Jarvis, W.R. (1996) The role of understaffing in central venous catheter-associated bloodstream infections. *Infect. Control Hosp. Epidemiol. 17*:150–8.

Gerber, S.I., Jones, R.C., Scott, M.V., *et al.* (2006) Management of outbreaks of methicillin-resistant Staphylococcus aureus infection in the neonatal intensive care unit: a consensus statement. *Infect. Control Hosp. Epidemiol. 27*:139–145.

Geva, A., Wright, S.B., Baldini, L.M., *et al.* (2011) Spread of methicillin-resistant Staphylococcus aureus in a large tertiary Neonatal Intensive Care Unit: network analysis. *Pediatrics 128*(5):1173–1180.

Harbarth, S., Sudre, P., Dharan, S., *et al.* (1999) Outbreak of Enterobacter cloacae related to understaffing, overcrowding and poor hygiene practices. *Infect. Control Hosp. Epidemiol. 20*:598–603.

Harris, A.D. and Thom, K.A. (2010) Control of antibiotic-resistant gram negative pathogens. In Practical Healthcare Epidemiology. Chicago: The University of Chicago Press.

Havill, N.L., Havill, H.L., Mangione, E., Dumigan, D.G., *et al.* (2011) Cleanliness of portable medical equipment disinfected by nursing staff. *Am. J. Infect. Control 39*:602–4.

Jackson, M., Chiarello, L.A., Gaynes, R.P. and Gerberding, J.L. (2002) Nurse staffing and healthcare-associated infections: Proceedings from a working group meeting. *Am. J. Infect. Control 30*:199–206.

Joint Commission. National Patient Safety Goals. http://www.jointcommission.org/assets/1/6/NPSG_Chapter_Jan2012_HAP.pdf Accessed on February 15, 2012.

Klevens, R.M., Edwards, J.R., *et al.* (2007) Estimating healthcare-associated infections and deaths in U.S. hospitals, 2002. *Public Health Reports 122*:160–166.

Morgan, D.J., Rogawski, E., Thom, K.A., *et al.* (2012) Transfer of multi drug-resistant bacteria to healthcare worker gloves and gowns after patient contact increases with environmental contamination. *Crit. Care Med. 40*(4):1045–51.

Muto, C.A., Jernigan, J.A., Ostrowsky, B.E., *et al.* (2003) SHEA Guideline for Preventing Nosocomial Transmission of Multidrug—Resistant Strains of Staphylococcus aureus and Enterococcus. *Infect Control Hosp Epidemiol 24*:362–386.

NICU Nursery Rooms and Areas—2.2–2.10.2.2 Space requirements. In: Guidelines for Design and Construction of Healthcare Facilities, 2010 edition.

Pessoa-Silva, C.L., Posfay-Barbe, K., Pfister, R., *et al.* (2005) Attitudes and perceptions toward hand hygiene among healthcare workers caring for critically ill neonates. *Infect. Control Hosp. Epidemiol. 26*:305–311.

Rupp, M.E., Adler, A., Schellen, M., *et al.* (2010) Hospital-Wide Assessment of Patient Room Environmental Cleanliness. Presented at the Fifth Decennial International Conference on Healthcare-Associated Infections, March 2010, Atlanta, Georgia.

Siegel, J.D., Rhinehart, E., Jackson, M., Chiarello, L. and the Healthcare Infection Control Practices Advisory Committee. (2007). Guideline for Isolation Precautions: Preventing Transmission of Infectious Agents in Healthcare Settings.

Snyder, G.M., Thom, K.A., Furuno, J.P., *et al.* (2008) Detection of methicillin-resistant Staphylococcus aureus and vancomycin-resistant Enterococcus on the gowns and gloves of healthcare workers. *Infect. Control Hosp. Epidemiol. 29*:583–589.

Thom, K.A., Johnson, J.K., Lee, M.S. and Harris, A.D. (2011) Environmental contamination because of multi drug-resistant Acinetobacter baumannii surrounding colonized or infected patients. *Am. J. Infect. Control 39*:711–5.

CHAPTER 4

Essentials of Epidemiologic Measures and Data Interpretation

MAHER M. EL-MASRI, RN, PhD. and DAVY TAWADROUS Bsc. MD (C)

This chapter will provide a general case study that highlights evidence based practice infection control data. The intent of the chapter will be to provide healthcare professionals with the knowledge needed to understand infection control research and data reports. Additional content will include the role of the advanced practice professional in the identification and investigation of an outbreak.

4.1. CASE PRESENTATION

Sally is a public health nurse who has been dispatched as a member of a healthcare team to investigate the spread of various infectious diseases in a rural community. Sally and her team realize that data on the prevalence, incidence, or risk factors of various diseases have not yet been determined. The local healthcare providers want to learn how to collect and analyze infection control data so they can identify outbreaks sooner and determine methods to better prevent infections in their community. Sally and her team agree to analyze the community's infection and immunization data and report their findings and teach local providers how to do the calculations. They also are asked to make some comparative analyses and come up with inferential conclusions as to the rate of disease and the effects of different risk or exposing factors. Sally and her team present the following data on infectious diseases in the community to the local providers:

1. The cumulative incidence of measles for the year 2011 was 25% and the incidence was 0.1 for the population.
2. The incidence of HIV in the community was stable at 2.0%

49

every year between 2010 and 2012. However, the prevalence of the disease increased from 1.8% in the year 2010 to 2.2% in 2012.

3. There is an increased risk for acquiring gastrointestinal illness if drinking well water in the northeast portion of the community (RR 1.9, 95% CI 1.01–3.61).

4. Farmers exposed to phenoxy herbicides had an increased risk for urinary cancers (HR 5.7; 95% CI 2.43–18.92).

5. The rate of ventilator-associated pneumonia rate reported from the local hospital is high among those who stayed in the ICU for 10 days or more (20%) and is low among those stayed in the ICU for less than 10 days (10%). These data yielded a relative risk of 2.0 (95% CI, 1.7–2.6), suggesting that ICU admission for 10 days or more increases the risk of ventilator-associated pneumonia by two times compared to those who are admitted for less than 10 days.

Considering the importance of proper understanding of epidemiologic principles for the Infection Control Practitioner, this chapter provides an overview of the major measures of disease frequency and disease-exposure association. It also provides a brief overview of statistical probability (*P.* value) and confidence intervals—two commonly reported indicators in hypothesis testing procedures. The Chapter also briefly discusses the issue of clinical versus statistical significance in epidemiologic research.

4.2. MEASURES OF DISEASE FREQUENCY

1. The cumulative incidence of measles for the year 2011was 25% and the incidence was 0.1 for the population.

4.2.1. Cumulative Incidence

Incidence is a very good measure of risk in epidemiology, including the study of infectious diseases. Cumulative incidence describes the number of *new* cases in an *at-risk population*, over a specific *time period* (e.g., a week, month, year, decade, etc.), and is intended to measure the frequency of individuals who develop disease Y from a population who is at risk for developing that disease. As the definition implies, cumulative incidence is calculated by dividing the number of *new cases* of disease Y in a population during a *specific period of time* by the total number of people *at risk for disease Y* in that population during the same period of time.

In the previous sentence, three important phrases were italicized, as they are essential to the understanding and calculation of cumulative incidence. Notice that the numerator in the calculation is strictly limited to *new cases* of the disease that occur during a specific period of time. Thus, pre-existing cases of the disease cannot be included in the numerator count. Also notice that the denominator includes all individuals in the population who are *at risk* of developing the disease during that same period of time. That is, individuals who already live with the disease and individuals who cannot conceptually have the disease are excluded from the denominator count. Finally, notice that the definition specifies the period of time in which the population is observed. Also notice that this time is equal for all individuals at risk for developing the disease, usually a year.

To illustrate cumulative incidence, let us assume that a researcher is interested in exploring the incidence of measles in a given community during a given calendar year. In the numerator, the researcher will include only *new cases* of measles that occurred in that community during that calendar year (pre-existing cases of measles at the beginning of the year are excluded). Further, the denominator will not include individuals who are not at risk of measles (e.g., individuals who already have the disease or those who are immunized against it). In other words, the denominator will comprise only the number of individuals who did not have a known diagnosis of measles at the beginning of the surveillance. Given that the surveillance was confined to a particular calendar year, you will start the count at the first day of that year and will stop it at the last day of the same year.

2. The incidence of HIV in the community was stable at 2.0% every year between 2010 and 2012. However, the prevalence of the disease increased from 1.8% in the year 2010 to 2.2% in 2012.

4.2.2. Incidence Rate (IR)

Cumulative incidence is a useful measure of the disease occurrence in a particular population at a specific period of time (e.g., mid-year). It is, however, based on the premise that all individuals in the surveillance were equally followed for the same period of time (i.e., assuming all individuals were observed for equal time intervals). However, sometimes we are faced with situations in which individuals are not equally followed up. This situation commonly arises in hospital surveillance studies whereby not everyone enters the surveillance at the same time (patients are surveyed as they are admitted). Further, individuals may be lost to follow-up, suffer from competing diseases, or they may die during their follow up period prior to developing the disease. When different individuals are followed for different times, our denominator must be adjusted to the sum of the units of time that each individual was at risk. Incidence calculated based on this understanding is called 'Incidence Rate' or "Incidence Density" and is often expressed in terms of person-years of observation. Figure 4.1 below illustrates the concept of person-time, showing that individuals in our surveillance contributed different times to the total follow up period. This is because some participants either started late in the surveillance (Participants 2 & 5), or because they either developed the outcome or were lost to follow up before the end of the six year surveillance period (participants 2, 3, 4, and 5). By summing each individual's surveillance time, we obtain a total of 20 observation years. This 20 observation-years obtained from the 5 participants in our example is equivalent to that of 20 individuals being observed for an entire year.

Knowing the person-time in any given study or surveillance, one can calculate the incidence rate using the following formula:

$$\text{Incidence Density} = \frac{\text{New cases of disease Y during a specified period of time}}{\text{Total person-time}}$$

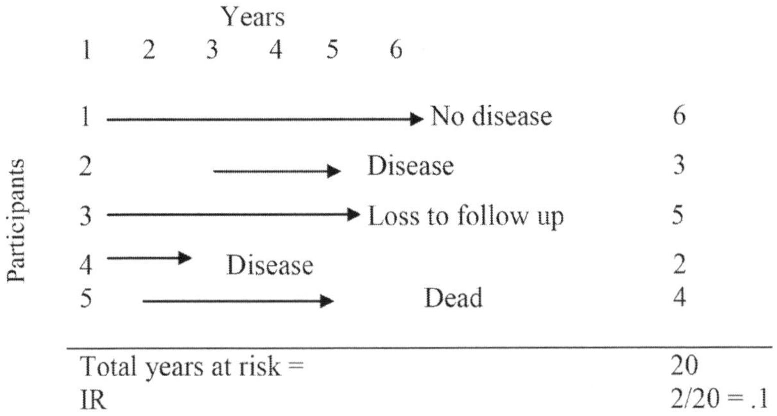

FIGURE 4.1.

Given that only 2 individuals in our surveillance developed the disease, we conclude that the incidence rate is 2/20 or 0.1. That is, one person develops the disease per 10 persons, per year. In other words, if we were to follow 10 people for one year, we would end up with one individual developing the disease during this year. Notice that if we were to calculate the cumulative incidence, we will get a different result that is somewhat larger 2/5 = 0.25 or 25%. This is because cumulative incidence does not account for the fact that individuals may contribute different time intervals to the follow up period.

4.2.3. Prevalence

While incidence informs us how fast a disease is spreading, prevalence informs us of how many people are affected by a disease. Specifically, prevalence describes the proportion of individuals in a population (old and new cases) that have the disease during a specific period of time.

Prevalence =

$$\frac{\text{Individuals with disease X during a specified period of time}}{\text{Total population during this specified time}}$$

Different measures of prevalence are used depending on the phenomena or disease of interest. Specifically:

- *Point prevalence* describes the number of individuals affected by a disease at *one point* in time. This approach to prevalence calculation is particularly useful in situations in which cases occur within a single day or very short period of time, such as in infectious outbreaks.
- *Period prevalence* is used to measure the number of individuals affected by a disease during a *period* of time (usually one year). This is a useful approach to measure the prevalence of relatively long lasting diseases such as Chlamydia infections from year to year.
- *Lifetime prevalence* describes the number of individuals affected by a disease at any time during their lifetime up to the time of assessment. Lifetime prevalence is very useful for policy makers who wish to learn about the overall spread of a given disease in a given population.

It is unfortunate that incidence and prevalence are sometimes confused and used interchangeably. The aforementioned discussion shows that they are different measures of disease frequency. Incidence tells us what is happening with regards to current spread of a disease, while prevalence tells us the overall spread of a disease (old and new cases) in a population (i.e., the total burden of disease). The two measures are, however, interrelated, and thus knowing both the incidence and prevalence rates in a population can provide meaningful information concerning the control and/or management of a disease. To help understand the relationship between incidence and prevalence, consider the epidemiologist's bathtub (Figure 4.2). Incidence is represented by the tap, which indicates the number of new cases of a disease. Both recovery and mortality are represented by water evaporation (recovery) and the drain (mortality), respectively, indicating cases leaving the bathtub. The water in the bathtub represents the prevalence of the disease at the time of assessment or surveillance. Together, all elements of the epidemiologist's bathtub are used to describe how the prevalence (overall burden of disease) is a function of the incidence (number of new cases), and recovery and mortality (number of cases being removed from the tub). So, is decrease in prevalence of a disease always a good thing? Using the epidemiologist's bathtub, we see that a decrease in prevalence may reflect a decrease in the number of new cases, recovery, or death from the disease. Therefore, unless we know the incidence of a disease, recovery rate from the disease, and the mortality associated with that disease, reduction in prevalence may not necessarily be a good thing. To illustrate this point, let us assume that the incidence of HIV in a given population was stable at 2.0% every year between 2010 and 2012. However, the prevalence of the disease increased from 1.8% in the year

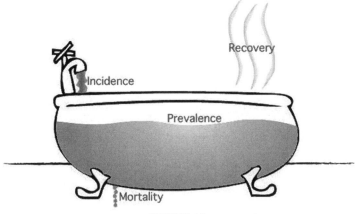

FIGURE 4.2.

2010 to 2.2% in 2012. Given that HIV has no cure yet, these statistics could be an indication that we are not only doing a good job in keeping the spread of HIV at bay, but we are also doing a very good job at improving the survival of HIV patients. Now, assume that the prevalence went down from 1.8% to 1.2%. In this case, we conclude that while we are doing a good job in controlling the incidence of the disease (remained stable at a low rate of 2.0%), we are not doing as well in treating those who already have the virus since the prevalence is decreasing as a result of increased mortality from HIV.

4.3. MEASURES OF DISEASE-EXPOSURE ASSOCIATION

In epidemiology, we are often interested in understanding the association between an exposing factor (i.e., exposure) and disease—that is, examining whether an exposure is associated with an increased risk of a given disease. This is often achieved by calculating the relative risk (RR), odds ratios (OR), or hazard ratio (HR). The selection of each one of these measures depends on the kind of available data and research design (beyond the scope of this chapter) used to generate the data. The following section explains each one of these measures with illustration. Notice however, that regardless of the measure, the goal is the same and that is to establish an association between exposure and disease.

3. There is an increased risk for acquiring gastrointestinal illness if drinking well water in the northeast portion of the community (RR 1.9, 95%CI 1.01–3.61).

4.3.1. Relative Risk

Risk is defined as the probability of disease occurrence in a cohort of people or a population. Thus, when we attempt to examine whether drinking contaminated water is associated with increased risk of gastrointestinal infections, we compare two risks: the risk of gastrointestinal infection among the cohort of individuals who drank the contaminated water compared to the risk of gastrointestinal infections among a comparable cohort of individuals who drank uncontaminated water. In this case, the risk of gastrointestinal infection in the exposed group (contaminated water drinkers) is reported relative to the risk of gastrointestinal infection in the unexposed group (uncontaminated water drinkers). The result of this comparison is called relative risk (Also known as

Risk Ratio). As health care providers, we use knowledge of the relative risk to make important decisions concerning patients' care and disease prevention and/or management. To calculate relative risk, we divide the risk of disease in the exposed group over the risk of disease in the unexposed group as demonstrated below, using the 2 × 2 cross tabulation table of the disease and exposure.

Exposure	Disease +	Disease −
+	a	b
−	c	d

$$\text{Risk Ratio} = \frac{\text{Risk of Disease in Exposed}}{\text{Risk of Disease in Unexposed}} = \frac{\dfrac{a}{a+b}}{\dfrac{c}{c+d}}$$

Relative risk or risk ratio (RR) is interpreted as follows:

1. RR = 1: the risk of the outcome in the exposed group equals that of the unexposed group, and thus there is no association between the exposure and outcome;

2. RR > 1: the risk of the outcome in the exposed group is greater than that of the unexposed group, and thus the exposure increases the likelihood of the outcome (exposure is deemed a risk factor—the larger the value of the relative risk, more likely the exposure is to bring about the outcome); and

3. RR < 1: the risk of the outcome in the exposed group is less than that of the unexposed group, and thus the exposure decreases the likelihood of the outcome (negative association—the smaller the value of the relative risk the more likely the exposure is to prevent the outcome).

While relative risk determines the *strength of the association* between an exposure and disease, attributable risk provides an estimate of *how much* of the disease is a function of the exposure. Consider the relationship between drinking contaminated water and gastrointestinal infection. While there is a positive association between the exposure and disease (i.e., RR > 1), attributable risk helps us determine how much of the incidence in gastrointestinal infection can be uniquely attributed to drinking contaminated water. It is important to note that not everyone who drinks contaminated water develops gastrointestinal infection. In addition, people may develop gastrointestinal infection due to factors other than drinking contaminated water (e.g., eating contaminated food and other unknown factors). These factors are referred to as background risks and are often present in both exposed and non-exposed individuals.

If we only consider the *exposed* group, we know that their total risk

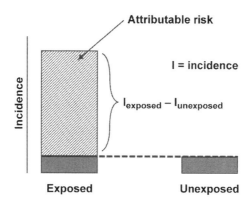

of disease is the sum of their attributable risk (risk due to exposure) and background risk (risk due to environmental or genetic factors). Thus, to determine how much of the total risk of the disease is actually due to the exposure, we calculate the arithmetic difference in the risk among the *exposed cohort* to the risk in the *unexposed cohort*. Note that attributable risk assumes causality, in that the level of absolute risk increase in the exposed group is solely due to the exposure.

$$\text{Attributable Risk}_{\text{Exposed}} =$$
$$\text{Incidence in Exposed} - \text{Incidence in Unexposed}$$

Conversely, the population attributable risk (PAR) considers how much of the disease incidence in the total population (composed of exposed and non-exposed individuals) can be attributed to the exposure. Similarly, we calculate PAR using the arithmetic difference of incidence rates in the total population and unexposed groups. This measure is particularly useful for determining the effect of an intervention on prevention of a disease in the total population.

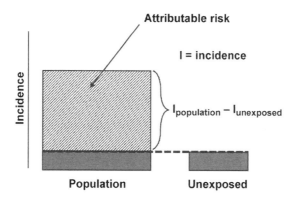

$$\text{Attributable Risk}_{\text{Population}} =$$
$$\text{Incidence in Total Population} - \text{Incidence in Unexposed}$$

4. Farmers exposed to phenoxy herbicides had an increased risk for urinary cancers (HR 5.7; 95% CI 2.43-18.92).

4.3.2. Hazard Ratio

If you recall from our earlier discussion, sometimes, individuals in a cohort are not uniformly followed for identical time periods due to the fact that some may (1) enter the study at varying times and (2) others may be lost to follow up for a variety of reasons. In instances like these, calculating the relative risk as described above will be naïve and misleading. This is because the different follow up times for individuals in the study must be accounted for by using a time-to-event analysis approach. It makes sense to think that one will not assume that the risk assessment of an individual who was followed for a single year is the same as that of another who was followed for 10 years. As a result, in instances like this one, it is important that we calculate the Hazard ratio instead of the relative risk, accounting for the different follow up times for each individual in the study.

Hazard ratio is calculated by dividing the incidence rate among exposed individuals (IR_{exposed}) by the incidence rate among the unexposed individuals ($IR_{\text{unexposed}}$), as demonstrated in Figure 4.3. A careful assessment of Figure 4.3 shows it presents the Incidence ratio (IR) for the exposed [Figure 4.3(a) and the non-exposed Figure 4.3(b)] groups. Notice that individuals in the example had varying observation or follow up times. Thus for each group, the IR was calculated by dividing the number of cases who developed the disease by the respective person-time for that group. The IR for the exposed group was then divided by the IR for the non-exposed to yield a hazard ratio of 1.2. This statistic can be interpreted to mean that the hazard of disease is 1.2 times (or 20%) higher in the exposed group than the non-exposed group.

Like relative risk, hazard ratios are interpreted as follows:

1. HR = 1: the rate or hazard of the outcome in the exposed group equals that of the unexposed group, and thus there is no association between the exposure and outcome;

2. HR > 1: the rate or hazard of the outcome in the exposed group is greater than that of the unexposed group, and thus the exposure

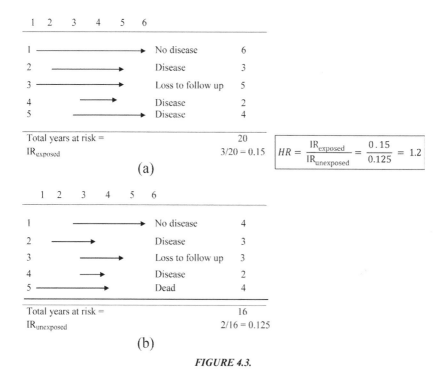

FIGURE 4.3.

increases the likelihood of the outcome (exposure is deemed a risk); and

3. HR < 1: the rate or hazard of the outcome in the exposed group is less than that of the unexposed group, and thus the exposure decreases the likelihood of the outcome (exposure is a protective factor).

4.3.3. Odds Ratio

At times, researchers may not have access to risk of disease and thus are unable to calculate the relative risk. It is also possible that the risk of disease is so rare (e.g., HIV/AIDS) that collecting data on such risk could take years and may be deemed unfeasible. In such instances, the use of odds ratios, which measure the association between exposure and disease, becomes an appealing alternative to relative risk or Incidence ratio. This is because calculation of odds ratios, in its simplest form, is based on comparing the exposure between a selected number of individuals who already have the disease to that of a matched group of individuals who do not have the disease (realize that now, unlike what we did when we calculated relative risk, we are going backward comparing diseased and non-diseased on their exposure).

To better understand odds ratios and their interpretation, it is important that we discuss the meaning of the odds first. The "odds" is best described as the probability of the event occurring in a group to it not occurring in the same group. In the Cross-tabulation table below, we can calculate the odds of exposure among the diseased cohort ($a + c$) as a/c. That is, the probability of being diseased and exposed (event) divided by the probability of being diseased but not exposed (no event); whereby exposure is the event. In the same cross tabulation, we can calculate the odds of exposure in the non-diseased cohort ($b + d$) in exactly the same approach to be "b/d". Now that we figured the odds of exposure in the diseased group (i.e., a/c) and the odds of exposure in the non-diseased group (i.e., b/d), we can divide the two odds to produce the odds ratio. The odds ratio is often used in Case-Control studies to determine the strength of association between an outcome or disease and the exposure, and results in statements such as: 'Given that this patient has outcome Y, they were X times more/less likely to have exposure Z.' The odds ratio is calculated as the odds of exposure among those who develop the outcome compared to the odds of exposure among those who do not develop the outcome.

$$\text{Odds Ratio} = \frac{\text{Odds of Exposure in Diseased}}{\text{Odds of Exposure in Non-diseased}} = \frac{\dfrac{a}{c}}{\dfrac{b}{d}} = \frac{ad}{bc}$$

Similar to risk ratios, we interpret the odds ratio (OR) as follows:

1. OR = 1: the odds of exposure among those who develop the outcome equals that of the unexposed group, and thus there is no association between the exposure and outcome;
2. OR > 1: the odds of exposure among those who develop the outcome is greater than those who do not develop the outcome, and thus those with the outcome are more likely to have the exposure (positive association); and
3. OR < 1: the odds of exposure among those who develop the outcome is less than those who do not develop the outcome, and thus those with the outcome are less likely to have the exposure (negative association).

Note that when prevalence of disease is low, the odds ratio can be used to approximate the relative risk or risk ratio. In fact, some researchers sometimes use OR and RR to mean the same thing.

5. The rate of ventilator associated pneumonia rate reported from local hospital is high among those who stayed in the ICU for 10 days or more (20%) and is low among those stayed in the ICU for less than 10 days (10%). These data yielded a relative risk of 2.0 (95% CI, 1.7–2.6), suggesting that ICU admission for 10 days or more increases the risk of ventilator-associated pneumonia by two times compared to those who are admitted for less that 10 days.

4.3.4. Statistical Inference

Fundamental to all statistical tests is hypothesis testing. Briefly, hypothesis testing involves determining whether one fails to reject the *null hypothesis* (H_o) or rejects the H_o in favor of the *alternate hypothesis* (H_a). A null hypothesis assumes that there is no significant difference or association between two variables or groups, while the alternate hypothesis suggests that there is in fact a difference or association between two variables or groups. Hypothesis testing is usually judged by the use of *P.* values and/or confidence intervals. This section will provide a conceptual review of these two principles with a special emphasis on their meaning and how they are used to judge whether or not one should fail to reject the null hypothesis (i.e., accept the null hypothesis) or reject the null hypothesis.

4.4. STATISTICAL PROBABILITY (*P.* VALUE)

The *P.* value, or the statistical probability value, refers to the probability that an outcome would essentially occur by chance. In epidemiologic and infection control research, it is often difficult to study an entire population of interest. Thus, researchers often conduct research using samples that presumably carry the attributes of their target population. Data obtained from these samples are then analyzed to make inferences or conclusions about the population. For example, a sample of 300 ICU patients may be selected to study the influence of ICU length of stay on the risk of developing ventilator associated pneumonia. Data obtained from these 300 patients could then be used to make conclusions about the association between ICU length of stay and ventilator associated pneumonia in all ICU admissions. However, given that sampling errors are almost inevitable, it is possible that these 300 patients may not be representative of ICU patients and could therefore yield results that may not necessarily be representative of, or applicable to, the entire ICU patient population. So, how do we know whether or not the results obtained from these 300 patients are true and are not a function of chance (i.e., may not be replicable or a true reflection of the state of affairs in the larger population)? For instance, if we observe that, in our sample, the rate of ventilator associated pneumonia is high among those who stayed in the ICU for 10 days or more (e.g., rate = 20%) and is low among those stayed in the ICU for less than 10 days (e.g., 10%), how certain are we that these observations and the absolute difference of 10% reflect reality? Is the rate of ventilator associated pneumonia truly higher after 10 days of mechanical ventilation? Is it possible that the observed difference between the two time periods are a mere function of chance due to a sampling error? The use of the *P.* value is an appropriate approach to answer an *a priori* question and here is how it works.

Researchers are expected to do a priori calculation (estimation) of their research sample so that they have enough participants to make meaningful conclusions about the population that the sample represents, whether committing type I error (falsely rejecting the null hypothesis) or Type II error (falsely accepting the null hypothesis). One important element of sample calculation is called the significance level or alpha (α). Alpha is usually decided by the researcher prior to conducting the research. It is usually assumed at 0.05, but can be 0.1, 0.01, or 0.001. When a researcher sets his/her alpha at 0.05, he/she is actually willing to accept that there is a 5% (0.05) chance that his/her decision to reject the null hypothesis (i.e., concluded a significant finding) could be wrong. A researcher who sets his/her alpha at 0.1 takes 10% (0.1) chance that his/her conclusion may be wrong. The alpha level is therefore like the scale against which researchers judge whether their obtained *P.* value (usually reported in the results) indicates the presence of statistical significance.

To illustrate the relationship between alpha and *P.* value, let us return to our example above and assume that two different studies attempt to compare the rate of ventilator associated pneumonia between those who stayed in the ICU for less than 10 days and those who stayed for 10 or more days. Now, assume that researchers in the first study set their alpha at 0.05, while researchers in the second study set their alpha at 0.1. After completing their analysis, both studies report identical relative risk of [(20%)/(10%)] or 2.0, indicating that those who stayed in the

ICU for 10 days or more were two times more likely to develop ventilator associated pneumonia than those who stayed for less than 10 days. Further, the *P.* values for both studies were strikingly similar at 0.07. Given that researchers in the first study set their alpha at 0.05 while those of the second study set their alpha at 0.1, the two teams will end up making different conclusions about these results! The *P.* value of 0.07 in the first study is higher than their preset alpha of 0.05. Thus, they will conclude that the observed mean relative risk of 2.0 is not statistically different from 1.0 (i.e., exposure is not a risk factor) and that the larger than 1.0 relative risk of 2.0 is only a matter of chance. However, the *P.* value of 0.07 in the second study is less than their preset alpha of 0.1, leading to reject the null hypothesis and conclude that the relative risk of 2.0 was statistically significant and that those who stayed in the ICU for 10 days or more were indeed two times more likely to develop ventilator associated pneumonia than those who stayed for less that 10 days. Notice however, that researchers in the second study were willing to take a higher percentage of chance (10%) than researchers in the first study (5%) and thus they could be having a higher percentage of error in their conclusion about their results. That is why alpha level shall be considered very carefully. The chance of conclusion error—that there is statistical significance (i.e., rejecting the null hypothesis)—increases as alpha increases. That is why an alpha of 0.05 is commonly accepted as the rule of thumb in epidemiologic, health, and psychosocial research.

4.4.1. Confidence Intervals

Confidence intervals (CIs) have a similar function to that of the *P.* value with regard to making inferential conclusions concerning the null hypothesis. However, the CI is among the most reliable indicators of hypothesis testing for reasons that we will explain toward the end of this section. A CI is the range of values within which we believe the population value being studied falls. CIs are reported in the results section of published research and are often calculated either for mean scores or for proportion data such as relative risk, odds ratio, and hazard ratio (calculation details are beyond the scope of this chapter). A 95% CI, which is the most common level used (others are 90% and 99%), means that if we were to sample a population, there is a 95% chance that the true polulation estimate is included between the lower and upper limits of the confidence interval.

To illustrate the 95% CIs for two proportions, let us return again to our ventilator associated pneumonia example. Recall that the risk of ventilator associated pneumonia among those who were admitted to the ICU for 10 days or more was 20%, while it was only 10% for those who were admitted for less that 10 days. These data yielded a relative risk of 2.0, suggesting that ICU admission for 10 days or more increases the risk of ventilator associated pneumonia by two times compared to those who are admitted for less that 10 days. However, this risk increase could be the function of chance unless its CIs suggest otherwise. Recall that a relative risk of 1.0 indicates that the risk of disease is the same between those who were exposed to the risk factor (e.g., ICU admission for 10 or more days) and those who were not (e.g., ICU admission less than 10 days). So, whenever we judge a relative risk (or, for that matter, an Odds ratio or Hazard ratio), we need to inspect its CIs. If the lower and upper boundary of the CIs include 1.0 [e.g., (0.82–3.6)], then we conclude that the results are not significant and that the relative risk of 2.0 is a function of chance or sampling error. If the range between the lower and upper bounds of the CIs does not include 1.0 [e.g., (2.1–3.5)], then we conclude that the results are significant—that the relative risk of 2.0 is real and that those who stay in the ICU for 10 days or more indeed have a risk of ventilator associated pneumonia that is twice as high as those who stay for less than ten days. Keep in mind however, that the narrower the CIs (the closer its lower and upper limits to each other), the stronger it is as an indication that the parameter value (population) is close to the estimate (sample value). In other words, narrow CIs indicate that the calculated result is a strong estimate of the true population value. A very wide confidence interval [e.g., (2.1–43.6)], should not be trusted and should raise red flags concerning the sample size. Now, let us assume that ICU length of stay was not measured using a cut-off point of 10 days. Rather, let us assume that it was measured using the mean ICU days. In this case, we can compare those who developed ventilator associated pneumonia and those who did not on their mean ICU days. However, in this case, we will be comparing the two groups using the CIs of the means instead of the CIs of proportion, as explained in the aforementioned section above. To illustrate the 95% CI of a mean value, say that ventilator associated pneumonia group had a mean ICU days of 15 days and the no-ventilator associated pneumonia group had a mean ICU days of 8.0 days. We can use our knowledge of these mean scores and their standard errors to calculate their respective 95% CIs to make a conclusion—whether the scores are different or not. However, let us first understand the CIs of the mean. Say that the CIs for the 15 days mean score was calculated to range between 10 and 17. This would be reported as: (mean, 15; 95% CI, 10–17), indicating that if other samples from the same population of ventilator associated pneumonia patients were generated and intervals for the mean of ICU days for these samples were estimated, 95% of the intervals between the lower limit of 10 and the upper limit of 17 would include the true mean of the population. Notice that the *width* of the CI range is very important in indicating how reliably the sample mean represents the population. If the range between the lower and upper limits of the CI is narrow—as it is in our example of 10–17—then the mean value of the sample is more likely to represent the true population. This is because the lower and upper limits of the CI will be very close to the mean value. However, if the range between the lower and upper limits of the CI is wide, say 6–32, then the sample mean of 15 is less reliable in representing the population. With such a range, it is possible that the population value could be as high as 32, which is far from the sample mean value of 15. In fact, as discussed earlier, a very wide CI in a study should be questioned because it indicates that more data should have been collected before any serious conclusions could be made about the population.

Now, let us consider how to use the CIs of two means to make an inference as to whether or not they are statistically different. Two mean scores are said to be statistically different if their respective CIs values do not overlap. This is because overlap of the CIs of two means suggests that they share the same plausible population value and that the true difference in their population scores is equivalent to zero. That is why some researchers provide the CI for the difference of two mean scores, instead of the CIs for the means themselves. In that case, the difference in the mean scores is said to be statistically significant if its CI does not include zero within the range of its lower and upper limits [e.g., (4.0–9.0)]. If it includes zero [e.g., (–1.0–5.0)], we conclude that the observed difference is not statistically significant.

To illustrate this point, let us return to our previous example of ventilator associated pneumonia and ICU days. Considering that the mean ICU days were 15.0 (95% CI; 10.0–17.0) for the ventilator associated pneumonia group and 8.0 (95% CI; 6–11) for the non-ventilator associated pneumonia group, we notice that the two groups have a difference of 7.0 days. The question becomes, "Is this difference of 7.0 days statistically significant?" Notice that the range of values between 10 and 11 in the first CI is included in the second CI. Thus, we concluded that there is an overlap between the two CIs and that the 7.0 days difference is not statistically significant from zero. Now, let us assume that the mean days score was 15 days (95% CI; 13.0–17.0) for the ventilator associated pneumonia group versus 8 days (95% CI; 6.0–9.0) for the non-ventilator associated pneumonia group. In this case, we see that the two CIs do not overlap—none of the values for the first CI are included in the range of values for the second CI. Thus, we conclude that the mean difference of 8.0 days is statistically significant from zero.

4.5. CLINICAL VERSUS STATISTICAL SIGNIFICANCE

Just because the results of an epidemiologic research study indicate that the results are statistically significant, one cannot always conclude that they are clinically significant. In some instances, the smallest of effect sizes can be statistically significant simply because the sample size was too large. To illustrate this point, let us say that a researcher conducts a study to compare the risk of pneumonia between those who receive oral Chlorhexidine rinse and those who receive standard oral rinse with water. Say that the relative risk was .98 (95% CI 0.91–0.99). In this instance we see that Chlorhexidine rinse is statistically better than oral rinse. However, considering the clinical significance of this result one sees that reduction in the risk of pneumonia was very trivial to carry any clinical significance. In fact, by flipping reference of these relative risks (1/.98 = 1.02), one concludes that those who rinse with water increase their risk for pneumonia by only 2% compared to those who rinse with Chlorhexidine—clearly there is very little clinical significance of this finding although it was statistically significant. Now consider that the study found that the relative risk was 0.32 (95% CI; 0.23–0.38). Clearly this is not just a statistically significant finding, but is also a clinically significant, showing a clinically significant reduction in the risk of pneumonia in patients who rinse with Chlorhexidine compared to those who rinse with water. Another indication of clinical significance is the concept of the Number needed to treat in randomized clinical trials. The Number Needed to Treat (NNT) is calculated as:

$$NNT = \frac{1}{|\text{Drug Event Rate} - \text{Placebo Event Rate}|}$$
$$= \frac{1}{|\text{Absolute Risk Reduction (ARR)}|}$$

To interpret the NNT, the value represents the number of patients that would need to be treated with the drug in order to prevent one bad outcome (i.e., the number needed to be treated for one patient to benefit from the treatment). The higher the value, the more patients we would need to treat with the drug to prevent a bad outcome and, therefore, the less effective the drug. Thus, it is not enough to look at the statistical significance of a study's results without considering their clinical significance by looking at indicators of effect size such as relative risk, odds ratio, hazard ratio, and NNT.

4.6. SUMMARY POINTS

- Measures of disease frequency: cumulative incidence, incidence rates and prevalence
- Measures of disease exposure: relative risk, hazard ratios, odds ratios and statistical inferences
- Statistical probability: confidence intervals
- Clinical versus statistical significance

4.7. REFERENCES

Gordis, L. (2009). *Epidemiology* (4th ed.). Philadelphia: Elsevier.

Lang, T. and Secic, M. (2006). *How to Report Statistics in Medicine: Annotated Guidelines for Authors, Editors, And Reviewers* (2nd ed.). Philadelphia: American College of Physicians.

Newton, R. and Rudestam, K. (1999). *Your statistical consultant: Answers to your data analysis questions.* Thousand Oaks, CA: Sage.

CHAPTER 5

Infection Control in Acute Care Settings

JEANNE HINTON SIEGEL, PhD, ARNP

Topics included in this chapter will highlight the transmission of a staph infection from one patient to another in a healthcare environment. Immediately following, general discussion about safe hand hygiene practices, engineering controls, new monitoring techniques and use of isolation practices will be discussed. An introduction to a variety of healthcare environments will be provided to highlight infection control practices or procedures in settings in which the advanced practice health professional may be employed. Additional content will include the responsibility of the advanced practice professional in public health and importance of reporting communicable diseases.

5.1. CASE PRESENTATION

Sarah is a recent graduate from a Bachelor of Science in Nursing Practice (BSN) in a large city. She was delighted when she landed a job on the step down trauma telemetry floor of a public hospital on the night shift. Sarah has now completed her 3 month new graduate orientation and 6 week orientation to the floor. As she reports to her floor she discovers that they are a little short staffed and that they will all have 7 patients per nurse on the 60 bed unit with only one nursing assistant. The charge nurse who serves as her mentor will also have a full patient load of 7 patients. Sarah's 7 patients include a 26 y/o male hit by a bus, a 16 y/o female post motor vehicle accident (MVA), a 65 y/o homeless woman who was found unconscious after an assault, a 77 y/o woman that fell in her home two weeks ago and fractured her hip, a 56 y/o male assault victim found intoxicated with numerous wounds including blunt force trauma to chest and abdomen, a 48 y/o woman who fell down a flight of stairs and sustained a closed humeral fracture, and 38 y/o male with multiple stab wounds sustained in a knife fight.

John P. is a 26 y/o male was hit by a metro bus while crossing the street 6 weeks ago. He sustained fractures of his pelvis, femur, tibia and fibula. He was unconscious on admission and was diagnosed with a closed head injury. He has spent 5 weeks in the intensive care unit on a ventilator with multiple episodes of hypoxia. He underwent multiple surgeries to repair the fractures and craniotomy to correct a large subdural hematoma. He is currently oriented only to name and is not following commands. He has been placed near the nursing station because he has attempted to get out of bed despite his inability to bear weight. He has multiple wounds requiring daily dressing including the pin sites, the craniotomy incision, and pressure ulcers. The sacral pressure ulcer is a stage 3 and infected with staph. aureus. His bilateral heel pressure ulcers are filled with eschar and will be debrided in the operating room tomorrow. Due to the Methicillin Resistant Staph Aureus (MRSA) infections in his wounds, John P. will be one of the last cases on tomorrow's schedule. This patient is currently on contact isolation.

Maggie B., a 16 y/o female, was involved in a MVA two weeks following her birthday and admitted through the emergency room two days ago with a fractured arm and pneumothorax. The chest tube is to suction drain significant amounts of clear serous drainage. She has significant bruising from the steering wheel and was not wearing a seat belt when the accident occurred. Her mother does not leave her side. In addition, a never-ending stream of high school friends is in to visit the young patient; frequently sitting on the bed and using the patient's bathroom. The day nurse has attempted to control the traffic, for infection control reasons, but admits she had to call security twice to enforce the visiting rules.

The homeless woman, estimated to be about 65 years old, is a Jane Doe; attempts to identify her have been unsuccessful. She was admitted with multiple injuries including contusions and a stab wound to the abdomen. She was severely hypotensive and underwent a laparoscopy with a resection of her small bowel secondary to the stab wound. She is confused and has already gone through what appears to be drug withdrawal. She has evidence of an IV drug abuse history with visible tracks on her arms. Admission drug testing was positive for opioids. The patient was also found to have active Hepatitis C and is HIV positive with a low CD4 count. Her wounds are all showing signs of infection. The wounds have been cultured and the results are pending. She was placed on contact isolation this morning for fear that she has MRSA in her wounds.

A 77 y/o woman, Katherine C., fell in her home two weeks ago and fractured her hip. Her level of confusion goes from totally confused and attempting to get out of bed without assistance to mildly confused and pleasant. She had an open reduction internal fixation (ORIF) of an intertrochanteric hip fracture and is currently bed bound. Attempts to get her in a chair or bedside commode have resulted in the patient becoming combative. She is incontinent of bowel and bladder. Her sacrum has evidence (Stage 1) of pressure ulcer development. She is not tolerating attempts to turn her every two hours. A low air-loss bed has been ordered and should be in place tomorrow. Her children are flying in from out of town to begin discharge planning to a nursing facility closer to one of their homes.

Sarah's fifth patient, Kevin K., is a 56 y/o male assault victim found intoxicated with numerous wounds including blunt force trauma to chest and abdomen. He is awake and alert and refusing to cooperate with the detectives investigating his beating. He is threatening to leave the hospital against medical advice. His doctors are concerned because he has signs of sepsis and have what is believed to be Community acquired MRSA in all of his wounds.

Kitty W. is a 48 y/o woman who fell down a flight of stairs and sustained a closed humeral fracture and is awaiting surgery tomorrow for an ORIF to set her arm. She is awake and oriented and is walking in the halls. Since she is the first case in the operating room tomorrow Sarah will need to have all of her preoperative orders complete so the patient will be ready for the operating room at 7 AM. This patient is stable except for the need of frequent pain medications.

Her last patient, Bill H., a 38 y/o male with multiple stab wounds sustained in a knife fight, has just arrived from the recovery room. Of all of his stab wounds only one is serious. An emergency laparoscopy repaired an abdominal stab wound. Despite the surgery the patient is stable, awake, and alert. Unfortunately, he also sustained multiple defensive wounds on his arms and several puncture wounds on his thighs. Each of these wounds has been cleaned and sutured.

This is not an unusual situation for newly minted registered nurses to find themselves—on the off shifts with insufficient staffing and limited resources. Most new nurses are hired on the night shift or 7PM to 7AM shift. This is a shift with few support staff, including limited resources in central supply, laboratory, transportation, housekeeping and pharmacy. The availability of protective equipment such as gloves, gowns and masks can be challenging if the units are not well stocked. The availability of nursing personnel to assist each other in turning and cleaning patients without contaminating themselves and their clothing and equipment is scarce. Healthcare providers' equipment and clothing can be formidable vectors for transporting infection from patients and surfaces to other vulnerable patients. Equipment such as stethoscopes, penlights, blood pressure cuffs, and digital thermometers have all been found to be contaminated and capable of transmitting infectious agents.

This registered nurse is facing the challenges of a labor-intensive assignment with minimal support systems and patients who are limited in their ability to help themselves. In addition, the confused patients are unlikely to understand the instruction given to them. This nurse will have several patients with transmission based precautions as well as standard precautions to remember and implement throughout her shift. Failure to adhere to the precautions, including gowns and gloves to protect her hands and clothing, could result in the transmission of a multidrug resistant organism (MDRO) to other patients with open or surgical wounds. The routine disinfection of equipment is necessary to prevent the spread of infection, especially when the same equipment is routinely used on multiple patients.

5.2. ESSENTIAL CONTENT FOR INFECTION CONTROL

HAIs are infections that patients acquire as a result of their hospitalization and treatment. These infections may be difficult to treat because of the increased antibiotic resistance found in hospitals today and can range from uncomplicated to devastating complications (CDC, 2012). HAIs have contributed to an increase in the cost of healthcare since it is estimated that 1 out of every 20 hospitalized patients will contract an HAI. The cost of treating HAIs has been estimated to range between $35.7 billion to $45 billion annually in direct inpatient hospitals (Scott, 2009).

The sacral pressure ulcer is a stage 3 and infected with *staph. aureus*. His bilateral heel pressure ulcers are filled with eshcar and will be debrided in the operating room tomorrow. Due to the Methicillin Resistant *Staph Aureus* (MRSA) infections in his wounds, John P. will be one of the last cases on tomorrow's schedule. This patient is currently on contact isolation.

Healthcare Associated Infections (HAIs) are a mounting threat to patient safety, increasing morbidity and mortality, and adding to the cost of acute care. Recent studies have estimated the incidence of HAIs at 5–15% of hospitalized patients, with complications related to HAI in 25% to 50% of intensive care patients (Pittet, 2005). The greatest challenges in preventing and controlling HAIs are implementing improved surveillance and multiple drug resistant organisms and emerging pathogens.

5.2.1. Surveillance

Surveillance, or a systematic collection, analysis, and interpretation of necessary data, is instrumental in improving patient outcomes (Pittet, 2005). As early as the 1980s, the Study for the Efficacy of Nosocomial Infections or healthcare associated infections (HAIs) (SENIC) project demonstrated that effective programs could reduce infections by 32% (Pittet, 20055; Haley, Quade, Freeman and Bennett, 1980). In addition, the hospitals without effective infection control programs showed an average increase of 18%. This project also found that between 25% and 50% of all nosocomial infections where attributable to a few patient care practices. The practices included use and care of urinary catheters, use and care of vascular accesses, therapy and support of pulmonary functions, surgical procedures, and appropriate use of hand hygiene and isolation. Not surprisingly, present day studies have found similar causes of infection.

5.2.2. Antibiotic Resistance

Since the appearance of MRSA, identified in the United Kingdom in 1961, multi-drug resistant organisms (MDROs) have become commonplace in the hospital and healthcare community (Siegel *et al.*, 2006; Boyce *et al.*, 2005). MDROs are defined as microorganisms, predominantly gram positive and gram negative bacteria, that are resistant to one or more classes of antimicrobial agents. Healthcare providers (HCPs) should not be misled because the names of certain MDROs describe resistance to only one agent (e.g., MRSA, VRE). These pathogens are frequently resistant to most available antimicrobial agents (Shlaes,

1997). The MDROs of greatest concern to healthcare facilities include methicillin-resistant *Staphylococcus aureus* (MRSA), vancomycin-resistant enterococci (VRE), multidrug-resistant (MDR) gram-negative bacilli (such as Enterobacter, *Klebsiella*, *Acinetobacter*, and *Pseudomonas species* and *Escherichia coli*), and vancomycin-resistant *S. aureus* (Siegel *et al.*, 2006).

Failure to adhere to the precautions, including gowns and gloves to protect her hands and clothing, could result in the transmission of a multidrug resistant organism (MDRO) to other patients with open or surgical wounds. The routine disinfection of equipment is necessary to prevent the spread of infection, especially when the same equipment is routinely used on multiple patients.

In most instances, MDRO infections have clinical manifestations that are similar to infections caused by susceptible pathogens. It is the inability to treat these infections as they overwhelm the body that becomes of greater concern. The options for treating patients with these infections are often extremely limited when conventional therapy is no longer effective. In addition to the increased morbidity and mortality, MDROs contribute to increased lengths of stay and hospital costs. Newly emerging pathogens have already begun and will continue to keep infection control practitioners very busy in this new millennium. These include several pathogens or prion-based illnesses, such as SARS and HINI (H5N1 or H7N7), that have invaded the acute care clinical settings (Pittet, 2005).

5.2.3. Potential Infection Outbreaks

HAIs are a major focus of patient safety efforts in acute care environments. Recently, infection preventionists (IPs) have begun to focus on the events leading to infectious outbreaks in the hospital environment. These outbreaks lead to closure and disinfection of entire units in addition to the treatment of the patients who have contracted the infections. One study by Reinhart *et al.* (2012) discovered that 289 out of 822 United States hospitals disclosed that they had incurred 386 outbreaks. Four organisms—norovirus (18%), Staphylococcus aureus (17%), Acinetobactor spp (14%), and Clostridium Difficile (10%)—comprised nearly 60% of the organisms implicated in the outbreaks (Rhinehart *et al.*, 2012). Of note, norovirus, which causes a "stomach flu" known as gastroenteritis, was responsible for 65% of unit closures in health care facilities. When evaluating an outbreak the IPs must consider the patient population, causative agents, possible causes and modes of transmission to assess the appropriate infection control measures (Rhinehart, 2012).

5.3. HAND HYGIENE

The most important intervention to prevent the spread of and to reduce the incidence of HAIs in the acute care environment is hand hygiene. Multiple studies have demonstrated that the hands of health care workers are a potent vehicle for the transportation and transmission of pathogens (CDC, 2012; Chou, Achan and Ramachandran, 2012). According to evidence gathered by the CDC (2002), HAI pathogens are transferred from patient to patient on the hands of health care workers (HCWs) when they are present on the skin of patients, or have been shed onto inanimate objects nearby and are picked up on the hands of HCWs. These organisms, if they are capable of surviving on the HCWs' hand for even a few minutes, are transmitted to another patient if the HCW omits either hand hygiene or inadequately performs hand hygiene. The contaminated hands can transmit the pathogen either directly to the patient or to inanimate objects that will come into contact with the patient in the healthcare environment. Hand hygiene includes a variety of methods for sanitizing the hand before and after patient contact. The most common include the use of soap and water, and products containing alcohol and chlorhexidine.

Sarah's fifth patient, Kevin K., is a 56 y/o male assault victim found intoxicated with numerous wounds including blunt force trauma to chest and abdomen. He is awake and alert and refusing to cooperate with the detectives investigating his beating. He is threatening to leave the hospital against medical advice. His doctors are concerned because he has signs of sepsis and have what is believed to be Community acquired MRSA in all of his wounds.

To address the lack of knowledge in health care about good hand hygiene practice, the Centers for Disease Control and Prevention's Healthcare Infection Control Practices Advisory Committee published comprehensive guidelines. The CDC reviewed that available evidence for methods and products used in hand hygiene and outlined the advantages and disadvantages of each. In 2002, the *Guideline for Hand Hygiene in Health-Care Settings: Recommendations of the Healthcare*

Infection Control Practices Advisory Committee and the Hand Hygiene Task Force were published in the Morbidity and Mortality Weekly Report (MMWR). This committee (Boyce, Pittet *et al.*, 2002) developed comprehensive guidelines for hand hygiene. One of the major recommendations were the use of waterless, alcohol based hand rubs as a preferred method for hand hygiene. Their analysis of the evidence determined that in most situations, alcohol-based rubs had superior efficacy in rapidly reducing bacterial counts on hands and ease of use by HCWs (Boyce, Pittet *et al.*, 2002). However, wearing gloves is not a substitute for hand hygiene for the prevention of HAIs.

The current hand hygiene guidelines developed and published by the CDC and the World Health Organization (WHO) are directed at improving the technique and compliance of hand hygiene in the health-care setting. These guidelines for hand hygiene in health-care settings provide HCWs with a review of research data findings regarding hand hygiene and hand antisepsis in health-care settings, and provide specific recommendations to promote improved hand-hygiene practices. These recommendations address both the process of sanitizing the hands and the adherence to the timing of hand hygiene. HCWs should practice hand hygiene at key points in time to stop the transmission of microorganisms. Briefly, all HCWs should practice good hand hygiene before and after patient contact; after contact with blood, body fluids, or contaminated surfaces before invasive procedures; and before and after removing gloves. Wearing gloves alone is not sufficient to prevent the transmission of pathogens in healthcare settings and some studies have found that the routine wearing of gloves decreases the compliance to hand hygiene guidelines (Fuller *et al.*, 2011).

The CDC (2002) guidelines indicate that hand hygiene with soap and water or use of hand antisepsis should always be the practice in the following situations: when hands are visibly dirty or contaminated with material or are visibly soiled with blood or other body fluids, wash hands with either a non-antimicrobial soap and water or an antimicrobial soap and water. If hands are not visibly soiled, use of an alcohol-based hand rub is appropriate for routine decontaminating of hands in all other clinical situations. HCWs should decontaminate their hands immediately before and after direct patient contact. Hands should be decontaminated prior to donning sterile gloves. Hands should be decontaminated before inserting indwelling urinary catheters, peripheral vascular catheters, or other invasive devices. HCWs should decontaminate their hands even if only simple contact with intact skin occurs when moving patients and taking vital signs.

If the HCW comes in contact with body fluids or excretions, mucous membranes, broken skin, or wound dressings, hand hygiene is necessary even if the hands are not visibly soiled and even if gloves are worn. To prevent spreading infection from one body area to another on the same patient, a HCW should decontaminate their hands if they move from a contaminated site of the body to a clean site during patient care activities. Since medical equipment is a source of contamination, a HCW must decontaminate their hands after handling. Always decontaminate your hands prior to and after wearing gloves (clean or sterile). In addition, the CDC (2002, 2012) recommends that HCWs wash their hands using soap and water before eating and after using a restroom.

The CDC has conveyed some special situations that apply to acute care. These include limiting the use of antimicrobial impregnated wipes, as they are not as effective as alcohol-based hand rubs or washing hands with an antimicrobial soap and water for reducing bacterial counts on the hands of HCWs (CDC, 2012). The use of hand hygiene with soap (non-antimicrobial or antimicrobial) and water in the presence of spore producing organisms such as Bacillus anthracis is recommended due to the limited efficacy of alcohol, chlorhexidine, iodophors and other antiseptic agents against these microbes (CDC, 2012; D'Antonio *et al.*, 2010).

The World Health Organization (WHO, 2012) has developed a program of education and teaching resources to simplify the steps to successful hand hygiene in the healthcare setting. This program includes handouts and posters that depict the five moments requiring hand hygiene and the appropriate step-by-step procedure for using rubs (gels) and hand hygiene (soap and water).

Adherences to the guidelines are affected by numerous factors. Researchers have observed that physicians and other HCW who are not nurses have lower compliance to hand hygiene guidelines. Other factors that affect compliance are gender, location (intensive care unit), weekdays versus weekends, and the wearing of gowns and gloves. Research is ongoing to look for interventions that can positively affect compliance and have a high level of sustainability over time.

Both the CDC and the WHO have invested enormous resources in the control of infections, including hand hygiene. Healthcare practitioners have available CDC- and WHO-developed educational programs, videos, posters, and web applications for use by hospitals and education programs. All of these programs can be accessed on the CDC and WHO websites. The websites' addresses can be found in the "Infection Control Resource Table" at the end of this chapter.

5.4. ENGINEERING CONTROLS

Healthcare providers exposed to bloodborne pathogens are at risk for serious and life-threatening illnesses. The CDC estimates that HCWs sustain nearly 600,000 percutaneous injuries each year involving contaminated sharps (CDC, 2012). According to the National Institute for Occupational Safety and Health (NIOSH, 2012), controlling exposures to occupational hazards such as infections and sharps injuries is the fundamental method of protecting workers from harm in the workplace.

A hierarchy of interventions beginning with elimination, substitution, engineering controls, administrative controls, and Personal Protective Equipment (PPE) can control exposures. The concept behind this hierarchy of interventions is that the control methods at the top of the list are potentially more effective and protective than those at the bottom. The goal is to eliminate the potential threat, if at all possible.

This registered nurse is facing the challenges of a labor-intensive assignment with minimal support systems and patients who are limited in their ability to help themselves. In addition, the confused patients are unlikely to understand the instruction given to them. This nurse will have several patients with transmission based precautions as well as standard precautions to remember and implement throughout her shift.

Elimination and substitution are the most effective interventions at reducing hazards, but unfortunately, they also tend to be the most difficult and expensive to implement in an existing process. It is important that all processes still at the development stage be evaluated for infectious hazards. At this stage of development, elimination and substitution of hazards may be inexpensive and simple to implement. Healthcare providers familiar with the infectious potential should be involved in the design and development of programs and procedures to eliminate or find substitutions for potentially infectious hazards. For an existing process, major changes in equipment and procedures may be required to eliminate or substitute for a hazard (NIOSH, 2012).

A 77 y/o woman, Katherine C., fell in her home two weeks ago and fractured her hip. Her level of confusion goes from totally confused and attempting to get out of bed without assistance to mildly confused and pleasant. She had an open reduction internal fixation (ORIF) of an intertrochanteric hip fracture and is currently bed bound. Attempts to get her in a chair or bedside commode have resulted in the patient becoming combative. She is incontinent of bowel and bladder. Her sacrum has evidence (Stage 1) of pressure ulcer development.

Administrative controls, which include rapid identification, early identification, and isolation of known or suspected cases, can help prevent the spread of pathogens from one person to another. Personal protective equipment that protects the skin, mucus membranes, eyes, and respiratory tract of HCWs are frequently used with existing processes where hazards are not particularly well controlled (NIOSH, 2012). The cost of administrative controls and personal protective equipment (PPE) programs may be relatively inexpensive in the beginning, but over the long term can be very costly to maintain. Because administrative controls and PPE require significant effort on the part of the individual HCW, they have also proven to be less effective than other measures.

When elimination and substitution are not viable options, engineering controls are used to remove a hazard or place a barrier between the worker and the hazard. The goal of engineering controls is to isolate or remove the bloodborne pathogen hazard from the workplace. In the acute care setting, the engineering controls will typically be independent of HCW interactions. Health care administration may balk at implementing these engineering controls because the start-up cost can be higher than the cost of administrative controls or personal protective equipment. However, operating costs are frequently lower over the long run and may eventually lead to cost savings in other areas. Examples of engineering controls commonly seen in hospitals today are sharps disposal containers, self-sheathing needles, safer medical devices such as sharps with engineered sharps injury protections, and needleless systems. Sharps are defined as any object that can penetrate the skin including, but not limited to: needles, scalpels, broken glass, broken capillary tubes, and exposed ends of dental wires (CDC, 2012; NIOSH, 2012).

Needleless systems are devices (connectors, tubing and injection ports) that do not use needles for the collection of bodily fluids or the administration of fluids or medications after initial venous or arterial access has been established (NIOSH, 2012). In addition, special sharp devices engineered to prevent injury currently are available. These devices sheath or retract a needle or sharp before and after use. The needle or sharp is automatically retracted from the injection/incision site. This engineering-designed feature takes the human element out of the equation; therefore the chance of injury is significantly reduced.

Engineering controls that can take out the potential for human error are more likely to protect the HCW (NIOSH, 2012). Additional examples of engineering controls in the healthcare environment include: Use of High-Efficiency Particulate Arresting (HEPA) filters to prevent airborne infections, Ultraviolet Germicidal Irradiation (UVGI) to kill infections on surfaces, and negative pressure in the care of patients with Tuberculosis to prevent the spread of infection within the confines of the hospital environment (NIOSH, 2012).

In addition to the controls discussed previously, OSHA's Bloodborne Pathogens Standard can be found at 29 CFR 1910.1030. This standard outlines what an employer must do to protect workers who are potentially exposed to blood or other potentially infectious material (OPIM). Any employee who could reasonably be expected to come in contact with blood or OPIM as a result of their regular duties is protected under this standard.

The bloodborne pathogens standard requires employers to establish a written exposure plan and update the plan yearly to reflect any changes in the plan during the previous year. Employers must implement standard precautions, identify and use engineering controls, identify and ensure use of work place controls, and provide personal protective equipment (PPE). In addition, employees should have input into the exposure plan. The plan must also clearly describe the steps to be taken in the event of an exposure to bloodborne pathogens. Blood borne pathogens include Hepatitis B (HBV), Hepatitis C (HCV), other hepatitis infections, Human Immunodeficiency Virus (HIV), Malaria, and other potentially infectious pathogens.

Body fluids, other than blood, have been implicated in the transmission of infections. These include cerebrospinal fluid, synovial fluid, pleural fluid, amniotic fluid, pericardial fluid, peritoneal fluid, semen, and vaginal secretions. In addition, any body fluid contaminated with blood or saliva and body fluids in emergency situations that cannot be recognized should also be considered infectious (CDC, 2007).

5.5. NEW MONITORING TECHNIQUES

Healthcare facilities are mandated by Center for Medicare and Medicaid Services (CMS), Joint Commission on Accreditation of Healthcare Organizations (JCAHO), and the Centers for Disease Control (CDC) to survey, tract, and report HAIs occurring in both inpatient and outpatient settings. The implementation of electronic health records (EHR) has

TABLE 5.1. *Employer Compliance to OSHA's Bloodborne Pathogens Standard.*

In response to concerns over healthcare worker exposures and the existence of newly developed technology which could increase employee protection, Congress passed the Needle Stick Safety and Prevention Act. This act directed OSHA to revise the bloodborne pathogens standards to assure that employers identify and make use of effective and safer medical devices. The revision became effective April 18, 2001 (OSHA, 2012).	
Employee Input	Employers are required to document, in the Exposure Control Plan, how they received input from employees. This obligation can be met by: • Listing the employees involved and describing the process by which input was requested; or • Presenting other documentation, including references to the minutes of meetings, copies of documents used to request employee participation, or records of responses received from employees. *Occupational Safety and Health Administration (OSHA) will check for compliance with this provision during inspections by questioning a representative number of employees to determine if and how their input was requested.
Exposure Plan	This is a written plan to eliminate or minimize occupational exposures. The employer must prepare an exposure determination that contains a list of job classifications in which all workers have occupational exposure and a list of job classifications in which some workers have occupational exposure, along with a list of the tasks and procedures performed by those workers that result in their exposure.
Employers must update the plan annually	To reflect changes in tasks, procedures, and positions that affect occupational exposure, and also technological changes that eliminate or reduce occupational exposure. In addition, employers must annually document in the plan that they have considered and begun using appropriate, commercially-available, effective safer medical devices designed to eliminate or minimize occupational exposure. Employers must also document that they have solicited input from frontline workers in identifying, evaluating, and selecting effective engineering.
Implement the use of universal precautions	Treating all human blood and OPIM as if known to be infectious for bloodborne pathogens.
Identify and use engineering controls	These are devices that isolate or remove the bloodborne pathogens hazard from the workplace. They include sharps disposal containers, self-sheathing needles, and safer medical devices, such as sharps with engineered sharps-injury protection and needleless systems.

(continued)

TABLE 5.1 (continued). Employer Compliance to OSHA's Bloodborne Pathogens Standard.

Identify and ensure the use of work practice controls	These are practices that reduce the possibility of exposure by changing the way a task is performed, such as appropriate practices for handling and disposing of contaminated sharps, handling specimens, handling laundry, and cleaning contaminated surfaces and items.
Provide personal protective equipment (PPE), such as gloves, gowns, eye protection, and masks	Employers must clean, repair, and replace this equipment as needed. Provision, maintenance, repair and replacement are at no cost to the worker.
Make available hepatitis B vaccinations to all workers with occupational exposure	This vaccination must be offered after the worker has received the required bloodborne pathogens training and within 10 days of initial assignment to a job with occupational exposure.
Make available post exposure evaluation and follow-up to any occupationally exposed worker who experiences an exposure incident	An exposure incident is a specific eye, mouth or other mucous membrane, non-intact skin, or parenteral contact with blood or OPIM. This evaluation and follow-up must be at no cost to the worker and includes documenting the route(s) of exposure and the circumstances. The employer must keep a sharps injury log that documents healthcare worker injuries that result from needles and sharps. A written policy and procedure for needle stick and/or sharps injury should be available in all healthcare facilities.

reduced the work of collecting the data. Prior to the use of EHR, the data was collected by chart review which was very time consuming and inefficient. With the newer documentation systems, the data is entered into a searchable database that allows for the retrieval and analysis of data in real time. This gives healthcare institutions rapid feedback on interventions aimed at preventing HAIs and Healthcare Acquired Conditions (HACs).

The technology to teach, reinforce, and monitor compliance to guidelines, isolation precautions and hand hygiene are also advancing with technology. The use of simulation laboratories and videotaping with playback to teach and reinforce skills followed by performance debriefing allows for correction of poor technique in a simulated environment. One study, Beam *et al.* (2011), used the technique and found that each of the 10 participants had at least one breach of the standard airborne and contact isolation precautions. This allows for further reinforcement prior to caring for patients.

Several studies have employed the use of 24-hour video monitoring to evaluate consistent adherence to hand hygiene, infection control, and isolation guidelines. These studies use the video to gather data, ensure interrater reliability, and to serve as a motivator for compliance.

Automated surveillance (AS) is a process for obtaining infection control data through the systematic use of medical informatics and computer science technologies. These technologies include data mining and hypothesis-based knowledge discovery. In data mining, mathematical and statistical techniques are used in large databases to discover patterns and relationships that can be used to classify and predict. Hypothesis—based knowledge discovery differs from traditional data mining by requiring someone to ask a purposeful question (Wright, 2008). The benefits of automated surveillance are obvious; time saved over manual data collection, reduced error potential, ease of access, and enhanced surveillance capabilities (Obenshain, 2004).

5.6. USE OF ISOLATION TO PREVENT THE SPREAD OF INFECTIONS

In 2007, "Guidelines for Isolation Precautions: Preventing Transmission of Infectious Agents in Healthcare Settings" was published. The Healthcare Infection Control Practices Advisory Committee (HICPAC) set forth guidelines for standard and transmission based precautions. Standard precautions are based on the principle that all blood, body fluids, secretions, excretions (except sweat), non-intact skin, and mucous membranes may contain transmissible infectious agents (CDC, 2007). These infectious agents can be transmitted to HCWs and other patients.

The use of standard precautions includes a group of infection prevention practices that apply to all patients, regardless of suspected or confirmed infection status, in any setting in which healthcare is delivered. When circumstances exist in which differentiation between body fluid types is difficult or impossible, all body fluids shall be considered potentially infectious materials and standard precautions used to protect the HCW and prevent the spread of the bloodborne pathogens.

Three categories of transmission-based precautions guidelines were developed by HICPAC to address infections in which the transmission of the infectious agent is not prevented by standard precautions. The three transmission-based isolation precautions are: Contact, Droplet, and Airborne Precautions. In the event that a pathogen has more than one route of transmission—for example severe acute respiratory syndrome (SARS) or coronavirus—more than one transmission-based precaution may be used. Even in the event that transmission-based precautions are used, standard precautions are always used. The use of transmission-based precautions can lead to potential adverse effects on patients due to the isolation. These isolation interventions, although necessary, can lead to adverse effects including anxiety, depression, perceptions of stigma, reduced contact with clinical staff, and delayed treatments (Abad *et al.*, 2010). Great care needs to be taken to minimize the adverse effects of isolation.

Contact precautions are intended to prevent transmission of infectious agents from one person to another by direct or indirect contact with the patient or the patient's environment. Contact Isolation is implemented when there is suspicion or laboratory evidence that an infection exists. Practitioners may also implement contact isolation if there is a presence of excessive wound drainage, fecal incontinence, or other discharges from the body that suggest an increased potential for extensive environmental contamination and risk of transmission (CDC, 2012). As with all types of transmission-based isolation precaution, a private room is optimal. If one is not available, consultation with infection control personnel is recommended to assess the various risks associated with other patient placement options (Siegel *et al.*, 2007).

HCWs caring for patients on contact precautions must wear a gown and gloves for all interactions that may involve contact with the patient or potentially contaminated areas in the patient's environment. It is important that HCWs put on PPE upon entering the room and discard the PPE before exiting the patient room in order to contain pathogens, especially those that have been implicated in transmission through environmental contamination (e.g., VRE, *C.difficile*, noroviruses and other intestinal tract pathogens; RSV).

Droplet precautions are intended to prevent transmission of pathogens with "large-particle droplets" (> 5 µm) spread through close respiratory or mucous membrane contact with respiratory secretions. These pathogens do not remain infectious over long distances in a healthcare facility; therefore, special air handling and ventilation are not required to prevent droplet transmission. According to the CDC (2012), the infectious agents for which droplet precautions are indicated include *B. pertussis,* influenza virus, adenovirus, rhinovirus, *N. meningitides*, and group A streptococcus (for the first 24 hours of antimicrobial therapy).

Patients who require droplet precautions should be in a single patient room. If a single-patient room is not available, infection control personnel should be contacted to assess the various risks associated with other patient placement options. These risks include the type of patient who can be safely cohabitated with the infected patient. In the event that a patient is in a room with more than one bed, it is important that a spatial separation of > 3 feet be maintained; drawing the curtain between patient beds is especially important for patients in multi-bed rooms with infections transmitted by the droplet route. HCWs wear a standard mask (a respirator is not necessary) for close contact with an infectious patient; the mask is generally donned upon room entry. If patients on droplet precautions must be transported outside of the room, the patient should wear a mask (if tolerated) and follow Respiratory Hygiene/Cough Etiquette (CDC, 2007). As with all patients on transmission-based precautions, the patient should only travel out of the room if absolutely necessary.

Airborne precautions prevent transmission of airborne infectious agents with droplet nuclei (< 5 μm) that remain suspended in air and remain infectious over long distances. The pathogens that require airborne precautions include rubeola virus, varicella virus, *M. tuberculosis*, and possibly SARS-CoV (CDC, 2007). Patients who require airborne precautions should be placed in an airborne infection isolation room (AIIR); that is, a single-patient room which is equipped with special air handling and ventilation capacity that meets the American Institute of Architects/Facility Guidelines Institute (AIA/FGI) standards for AIIRs. These requirements include a monitored negative pressure relative to the surrounding area, 12 air exchanges per hour for new construction and renovation and 6 air exchanges per hour for existing facilities, and air exhausted directly to the outside or recirculated through HEPA filtration before return (CDC, 2007). Some states require such rooms in hospitals, emergency departments, and nursing homes that care for patients with *M. tuberculosis*. In addition, a respiratory protection program that includes education about use of respirators, fit testing, and user seal checks is required in any facility with AIIRs. HCWs caring for patients placed on airborne precautions should always wear a mask or respirator that should be donned prior to entering the room. Whenever possible, the CDC (2007) recommends that non-immune HCWs should not care for patients with vaccine-preventable airborne diseases (e.g., measles, chickenpox, and smallpox) even though the patient is isolated due to the increased risk of the HCW contracting the illness.

If airborne precautions cannot be implemented due to limited resources the best course of action is to mask the patient and place the patient in a private room with the door closed. All HCWs should be provided a N95 or higher level respirator. If respirators are not available, masks for HCW will reduce the likelihood of airborne transmission until the patient is either transferred to a facility with an AIIR or returned to the home environment, as deemed medically appropriate (CDC, 2007).

In order to accurately diagnose many infections, a laboratory culture and sensitivity (C&S) is required for diagnosis and antibiotic sensitivity. The turnaround for these tests is often 2 or more days. In order to protect the HCWs and other patients, transmission-based precautions must be implemented while the healthcare team awaits the results of these tests. Implementation of appropriate Transmission-Based Precautions at the time a patient develops symptoms or signs of a transmissible infection, or upon arrival at a healthcare facility for care, greatly reduces transmission opportunities while awaiting the test results. While it is not possible to identify prospectively all patients needing transmission-based precautions, certain clinical syndromes and conditions carry a sufficiently high risk to warrant their use empirically while confirmatory tests are pending.

Termination of transmission-based precaution varies depending on the natural progress of the illness and/or the risk for infecting HCWs or other patients. Infectious viral pathogens have a predictable time frame with recognizable stages—for example, the onset of fever and the defervescence that marks the infectious nature of the illness. For most infectious diseases (chicken pox, measles, influenza), this duration reflects known patterns of persistence and shedding of infectious agents. Once the patient is no longer in an infectious state the precautions can be discontinued. Other illnesses require testing before precautions are removed. For other diseases, (e.g., *M. tuberculosis*) state laws and regulations and healthcare facility policies may dictate the duration of precautions (CDC, 2007). In immune-compromised patients, viral shedding can persist for prolonged periods of time (many weeks to months) and transmission may occur during that time. In order to prevent transmission, the duration of contact and/or droplet precautions may be prolonged for many weeks.

5.7. REVIEW OF HEALTHCARE ENVIRONMENTS

The challenges of infection control and prevention have some unique needs in different health care environments. These areas include but are not limited to Oncology/Hematology, intensive care units (ICUs) and burn units. Nurses must consider the vulnerability of the host and increased risk for infection in these areas. Additionally, there may be a need to implement protective isolation (PI) in patients with severely compromised immune systems.

5.7.1. Oncology/Hematology Units

Bacterial infections are a major cause of morbidity and mortality in cancer and hematology patients who are neutropenic. Protective isolation (PI) is often necessary to protect the patients from infections of HCWs and visitors. The nurse's role in educating the patient and the family on precautions necessary to prevent transmission of infection to neutropenic patients is pivotal in managing infection risk. Neutropenia is an abnormally low level of neutrophils, a type of white blood cell that helps fight infection. Neutrophils help fight infection by destroying harmful bacteria and fungi (such as yeast) that invade the body. Patients and staff can decrease the risk of infection by strict adherence to the prevention guidelines, hand hygiene, and personal hygiene. The environment should be routinely disinfected.

> Her last patient, Bill H., a 38 y/o male with multiple stab wounds sustained in a knife fight, has just arrived from the recovery room. Of all of his stab wounds only one is serious. An emergency laparoscopy repaired an abdominal stab wound. Despite the surgery the patient is stable, awake, and alert. Unfortunately, he also sustained multiple defensive wounds on his arms and several puncture wounds on his thighs. Each of these wounds has been cleaned and sutured.

Close monitoring of the patient for signs and symptoms of onset of infection is important to ensure early intervention. Preventative measures such as prophylactic antibiotics and vaccines should be administered when appropriate for patients at risk. Recommended vaccinations include Influenza, Pneumococcal, Meningococcal, and Haemophilus Influenzae Type B (Wiwanitkit, 2010).

5.7.2. Intensive Care Units

In the fast-paced, intervention-intensive delivery of care in the ICU, basic nursing skills and knowledge are a key to preventing HAIs in the critically ill patient (Vandijck *et al.*, 2010). The basics of hand hygiene and standard and transmission-based precautions are instrumental in preventing the development of HAI in the ICU. The ICU, based on the acuity of the patient, uses a variety of high technology, invasive interventions to treat the critically ill patient. In addition, immunosuppressive and broad-spectrum antibiotics are routinely used in the ICU (Vandijck *et al.*, 2010; Blot, 2008), making the ICU patient more susceptible to HAIs.

Compliance to the CDC evidence-based recommendations to prevent the transmission of pathogens has been shown to decrease the incidence of HAIs (Labeau *et al.* 2009). The greatest challenge in the ICU is to assure compliance to these recommendations. Unfortunately, knowledge and compliance to these recommendations has been demonstrated to be very poor (Labeau *et al.*, 2009). Interventions that reeducate and reinforce compliance will decrease the development of HAIs in the intensive care unit. Examples of interventions that can improve compliance include education programs, visible reminders (posters), easy access to hand hygiene and isolation supplies, multidisciplinary collaboration and responsibility, implementation of care bundles, and staff participation in implementation (Vandijck *et al.*, 2009).

5.7.3. Burn Units and Burn Centers

Every year approximately 450,000 burn injuries occur in the United States resulting in 45,000 hospital admissions to a burn unit or burn center for treatment (ABA, 2012). Even though the survival of burn victims has improved over the past several decades thanks to advances in medical care, burn patients are at greater risk for infection related to their loss of protective skin, the body's first line of defense against infection. In addition, extended stays in the hospital expose them to HAIs and invasive procedures that increase the likelihood of systemic infection (Hodle *et al.*, 2006). Infection remains the leading causes of morbidity and mortality in burn patients (ABA, 2012).

Burns, also called thermal injury, are a common form of trauma requiring immediate specialized hospital or burn center care to minimize morbidity and mortality (Ralfa and Tredget, 2009). The total body surface area (> 30%), amount of full thickness burn, and prolonged open wounds or delayed treatment influence the morbidity and mortality from burn injuries (Ralfa and Tredget, 2009). The sources of the wound infections can originate from the patient's own normal flora (endogenous) or from environmental exposure (exogenous). In the burn units and ICUs, the most common transmission is from direct or indirect contact with the contaminated hands of HCW or the equipment. The equipment can include hydrotherapy equipment, treatment areas, and hospital beds.

Burn units are forever vigilant to prevent outbreaks of cross-colonization and infection. The staff use culturing and surveillance to monitor the infection rates, and identify trends looking for any change that might require intervention to prevent an outbreak. In order to prevent these outbreaks, specialized infection control measures are used in burn units including surveillance cultures, cohort patient care teams, strict enforcement of patient and staff hygiene, increased availability of hand hygiene (alcohol based) products, and the monitoring of antibiotic use and antibiotic susceptibility (Ralfa and Tredget, 2009). The use of isolation rooms and strict barrier precautions while delivering care to burn patients is necessary to prevent cross contamination of the wounds.

5.8. ADVANCED PRACTICE PROFESSIONALS' ROLES IN PUBLIC HEALTH

When an advanced practice nurse steps into the role of primary care and/or the coordinator of care in the acute care setting, the practitioner assumes responsibility for diagnosis, treatment, and follow up of active and potential infections. The practitioner also has an obligation to protect others from contracting transmittable infections. This is done by following appropriate isolation procedures and notifying the DOH of potentially communicable diseases. Individual advanced practice organizations have developed guidelines for infection control in their area of expertise. In addition, these responsibilities are outlined in the organization's nursing scope of practice.

5.8.1. Reporting Communicable Diseases

The reporting of communicable diseases encountered by a health care provider is extremely important. Advanced Nurse Practitioners (ANPs) serve in a variety of fields as the primary healthcare provider. Health care providers, or an employee of a school, state institution, laboratory or infection control institution that become aware of a diagnosed communicable disease, should alert the proper authorities as soon as possible. The report should be made to the local health department where the infected individual resides within 24 hours of diagnosis. It is especially important to notify the local Department of Health (DOH) if the disease requires quarantining the carrier. Every state has their individual DOH that requires healthcare practitioners to report communicable diseases. ANPs are required to have the knowledge and diagnostic capabilities to assess, treat, and report these illnesses. Each ANP should be aware of the rules and regulations that apply in their state and the diseases that require reporting.

In order to report a patient diagnosed with a reportable communicable disease, a NP will contact the DOH in the county where the patient lives. Be sure to gather the necessary information including the patient's full name, address, telephone numbers, sex, race, birth date, ethnicity, social security number and diagnosis. It is also necessary to indicate if the individual is pregnant. Have available the types of tests completed to attain the diagnosis. In addition, the practitioner should be sure to provide collection date and treatments provided. The laboratory and doctor's name must also be listed in the communicable disease report. When in doubt, the practitioner should check with their county or state website to get specifics on reporting procedures. Advanced level practitioners should not assume the physician or the lab has made the disease report.

Practitioners in the general practice area and the emergency room are in a unique position to observe when a cluster of patients are being seen for a similar complaint or constellation of symptoms. In addition to individual case reports, any unusual or group presentation of illness that may be of public concern should be reported to the local health authority by the most expeditious means. This cluster should be reported whether or not the illness is included in the list of diseases officially reportable in the particular locality. The practitioner should report this whether it is a well-known identified disease or an indefinite or unknown clinical entity. Preventing the spread in the community requires timely intervention and surveillance.

5.8.2. Infection Preventionist—Advanced Practice

The Association for Practitioners in Infection Control and Epidemiology (APIC) has recently completed its competency model for the Infection Preventionist (IP). This model has at its core the practices and principles of safety science, with an emphasis on patient safety. This expanded model will lead to a certification to accompany the IP role. The Advanced Practice Nurses will be experts in the area of surveillance, infection prevention and control, and precautions necessary to prevent transmission of infections. They will be instrumental in the ongoing research in preventing HAIs.

A recent addition to the proposed interventions for improving knowledge and compliance to infection control polices and guidelines are the required implementation of Certification in Infection Control (Pogorzelska *et al.*, 2012). In their study describing the use of infection control policies aimed at reducing Multi-drug resistant organisms (MDRO) and Clostridium difficile in the State of California and assessing various infection related outcomes, the authors found that hospitals participating in the Institute for Healthcare Improvement (IHI) guidelines and reporting the presence of an infection control director (certified in infection control) had significantly lower rates of Methicillin Resistant Staphylococcus Aureus (MRSA) blood stream infections (BSI).

Another expanding role for nurses is a Masters in Science degree (MSN) as a Clinical Nurse Specialist in either infection control (IC-CNS) or infectious disease (ID-CNS). In addition, the ANP in infectious disease (ID-ANP) was developed. The role of the IC-CNS will provide focused expertise in infection control within and across clinical healthcare settings (Gail *et al.*, 2004). Providing focused expertise in infectious disease in clinical settings will be the scope of the ID-CNS. Additionally, Nurse practitioners (ID-ANP) is directed toward primary care with the scope of managing a group of patients with microbial, opportunistic, or superimposed acute or chronic disease (Gail *et al.*, 2004).

In summary, controlling infections in the acute healthcare environment is a complicated procedure requiring a healthcare team consisting of the practitioner, nurses, infection control expert, and administration. This team must work together to educate and implement the recommended guidelines developed to curb the spread of HAIs. The guidelines are only effective if compliance of HCWs is consistent. Researchers continue to look for new and inventive methods to increase and monitor compliance.

5.9. REFERENCES

Abad, C., Fearday, A. and Safdar, N. (2010). Adverse effects of isolation in hospitalized patients: a systematic review. *Journal of Hospital Infection, 76*(2): 97–102.

American Burn Association. (2012). Burn Incidence and Treatment in the United States: 2011 Fact Sheet. Retrieved online May 30, 2012 from http://www.ameriburn.org/resources_factsheet.php

Beam, E.L., Gibbs, S.G., Boulter, K.C., Beckerdite, M.E. and Smith, P.W. (2011). A method for evaluating health care workers' personal protective equipment technique. American *Journal of Infection Control, 39*(5): 415–420. doi:10.1016/j.ajic.2010.07.009.

Blot, S. (2008). Limiting the attributable mortality of nosocomial infections and multidrug resistance in the intensive care units. *Clinical Microbiology and Infection.*
14: 5–13.

Boyce, J.M., Pittet, D., *et al.* (2002). Guideline for hand hygiene in health-care settings:
recommendations of the Healthcare Infection Control Practices Advisory Committee and the HICPAC/SHEA/APIC/IDSA Hand Hygiene Task Force. *Morbidity and
Mortality Weekly Report, 51*(RR16):1–45.

Boyce, J.M., Cookson, B., and Christiansen, K. (2005). Methicillin-resistant Staphylococcus aureus. *Lancet Infectious Diseases, 5*: 653–663.

Center for Disease Control. (2007). Guidelines for Isolation Precautions: Preventing
Transmission of Infectious Agents in Healthcare Settings. Retrieved online May 21,
2012 from http://www.cdc.gov/hicpac/2007IP/2007ip_fig.html

Center for Disease Control. (2012). Healthcare-associated infections (HAIs). Retrieved
online 04/30/2012 from http://www.cdc.gov/HAI/burden.html.

Centers for Disease Control (CDC), 2012. Hand Hygiene Basics. Retrieved on April
14, 2012 from http://www.cdc.gov/handhygiene/Basics.html.

Chou, D.T., Achan, P. and Ramachandran, M. (2012). The World Health Organization's '5 moments of hand hygiene': The scientific foundation. *Journal of Bone &
Joint Surgery, British Volume, 94*(4): 441–445.

D'Antonio, N., Rihs, J.D., Stout, J.E. and Yu, V.L. (2010). Revisiting the hand wipe
versus gel rub debate: Is a higher-ethanol content hand wipe more effective than an
ethanol gel rub? *American Journal of Infection Control, 38*(9): 678–682.

Fuller, C., Savage, J., Besser, S., Hayward, A., Cookson, B., Cooper, B. and Stone,
S. (2011). "The dirty hand in the latex glove": A study of hand hygiene compliance when gloves are worn. *Infection Control & Hospital Epidemiology, 32*(12):
1194–1199.

Gail, C., Field, K.W., Simpson, T. and Bond, E.F. (2004). Clinical nurse specialist and
nurse practitioners: Complementary roles for infectious disease and infection control. *American Journal of Infection Control 32*: 239–42.

Haley, R.W., Quade, D., Freeman, H.E. and Bennett, J.V. (1980). The SENIC Project.
Study on the efficacy of nosocomial infection control (SENIC Project). *American
Journal of Epidemiology, 111*(5): 472–85.

Hodle, A.E., Richter, K.P. and Thompson, R.M. (2006). Infection control practices in
U.S. burn units. *Journal of Burn Care Research 27*: 142–151.

Klevens, R.M. (2002) Estimating health care-associated infections and deaths in U.S.
hospitals, 2002. *Public Health Reports 22*: 160–66.

Labeau, S.O., *et al.* (2009). Centers for Disease Control and Prevention guidelines for
preventing central venous catheter-related infections: Results of a knowledge test
among 3405 European intensive care nurses. *Critical Care Medicine, 3*: 320–323.

National Institute for Safety for Occupational Safety and Health (NIOSH). (2012). Engineering Controls. Retrieved on 05/1/2012 from http://www.cdc.gov/niosh/topics/
engcontrols/.

Obenshain, M.K. (2004). Application of data mining techniques to healthcare data.
Infection Control and Hospital Epidemiology 25: 690–5.

Pittet, D. (2005). Infection control and quality health care in the new millennium. *American Journal of Infection Control, 33*: 258–67.

Pogorzelska, M., Stone, P., W., & Larson, E., L. (2012). Certification in infection control matters: Impact of infection control department characteristics and policies
on rates of multidrug-resistant infections. *American Journal of Infection Control,
40*(2): 96-101. doi:10.1016/j.ajic.2011.10.002

Ralfa, K. and Tredget, E.E. (2009). Infection control in the burn unit. *Burns 37*: 5–15.

Rhinehart, E., Walker, S., Murphy, D., O'Reilly, K., & Leeman, P. 2012. Frequency of outbreaks investigations in US hospitals: Results of an national survey of infections. *American Journal of Infection Control 40*: 2–8.

Scott II, D.R. (2009) The Direct Medical Costs of Healthcare-Associated Infections in U.S. Hospitals and the Benefits of Prevention. CDC DHQP (March 2009).

Shlaes, D.M., Gerding, D.N., John, J.F., Jr., *et al.* (1997). *Infect Control Hosp Epidemiol, 18*: 275–291.

Siegel J.D., Rhinehart, E., Jackson, M., Chiarello, L. and the Healthcare Infection Control Practices Advisory Committee. (2006). Management of multidrug?resistant organisms in healthcare settings, 2006. Available at: http://www.cdc.gov/hicpac/mdro/mdro_0.html. 2006. Accessed June1, 2012.

Siegel, J.D., Rhinehart, E., Jackson, M., Chiarello, L., and the Healthcare Infection Control Practices Advisory Committee. (2007) Guideline for Isolation Precautions: Preventing Transmission of Infectious Agents in Healthcare Settings. Available at: http://www.cdc.gov/ncidod/dhqp/pdf/isolation2007.pdf Accessed June 1, 2012.

Vandijck, D.M., Labeau, S.O., Vagelaers, D.P., and Blot, S.I. (2010). Prevention of nosocomial infections in the intensive care unit. Position paper delivered at the British Association of Critical Care Association International Conference September 14–16, 2009.

Wiwanitkit, V. (2010). Important vaccines used as tools for tertiary prevention in oncology patients. *Indian Journal of Cancer, 47*(3): 339–43.

Wright, M.O. 2008. Automated surveillance and infection control: Toward a better tomorrow. *American Journal of Infection Control 36*(S1): 1–6.

World Health Organization. 2012. Five Moments for Hand Hygiene in Healthcare. Retrieved 05/18/2012 online from http://www.who.int/gpsc/tools/Five_moments/en/index.html

TABLE 5.2. Infection Control Resource Table.

Resource Title	Summary	Author	Web Reference
Toolkit to help control and prevent Norovirus Outbreaks in Healthcare Settings	CDC recently released a toolkit for health-care professionals who may have to deal with possible or confirmed outbreaks of Norovirus gastroenteritis	CDC	www.aafp.org/news-now/health-of-the-public/20120118norovirus.html
Bloodborne Pathogen Standards (OSHA)	Detailed requirements and compliance guidelines for OSHA 29CFR 1910.1030.	United States Department of Labor – Occupational Safety & Health Administration	www.osha.gov/pls/oshaweb/owadisp.show_document?p_table=STANDARDS&p_id=10051
Five Moments for Hand Hygiene—available in English and French	The Five Moments align with the evidence base concerning the spread of HAI but it is interwoven with the natural workflow of care and is designed to be easy to learn, logical and applicable in a wide range of settings. Includes posters and handouts on the proper steps of hand hygiene.	World Health Organization	http://www.who.int/gpsc/tools/Five_moments/en/index.html
Controlling exposures to occupational hazards	Hierarchy of controlling Occupational Hazards: • Elimination • Substitution • Engineering Controls • Administrative Controls • Personal Protective Equipment	National Institute for Occupational Safety and Health (NIOSH)	http://www.cdc.gov/niosh/programs/eng/
2007 Guideline for Isolation Precautions: Preventing Transmission of Infectious Agents in Healthcare Settings	HICPAC 2007 Isolation Prevention Guidelines	CDC HICPAC	http://www.cdc.gov/hicpac/2007IP/2007ip_fig.html

CHAPTER 6

Infection Control in Critical Care Settings

MARY WYCKOFF Phd., RN ANP

This chapter will begin with a case study exploring a multi-system failure patient with a hospital-acquired infection. Topics will include the infection control principles associated with the insertion of invasive vascular lines, dressing changes, and specific procedures completed by critical care nurse practitioners or physician assistants that work in the area.

6.1. CASE PRESENTATION

NW is a 34 year patient who was admitted into the Intensive Care Unit (ICU) due to fever, chills and hypotension. He arrived in the emergency department (ED) with complaints of nausea, vomiting and fever with general malaise. He said the onset was within the last 48 hours. His past medical history included diabetes, juvenile onset age 11, moderately controlled with insulin, renal insufficiency, and asthma. He had no past surgical history. His current medications include regular insulin, lantus, albuteral, and advair.

Upon admission to the ICU, Jan, the acute care nurse practitioner (ACNP), reviewed the laboratory data and completed a thorough review of the patient. Although his white blood cell count (WBC) was 2.4 mm^3, his temperature of 35.6 centigrade was concerning. He had difficulty breathing with an oxygen saturation of 92% on a 50% non-rebreather mask and his respirations were mildly labored. He had diminished breath sounds throughout and his chest radiograph showed consolidation in the right lower lobe. His urine was cloudy and his urinalysis showed greater than 50 WBCs. His heart rate was 112, sinus tachycardia, and his blood pressure ranged between 92/50–120/80 mmhg. The rest of his physical exam was normal. However, since he was at risk for MRSA, all blood and urine cultures were obtained as well as a nasal swab for MRSA.

Jan was concerned that NW was at risk for a significant septic episode and needed to provide appropriate broad spectrum antibiotics without placing him at risk for further renal failure. Based upon the ICU's antibiogram, the medication of choice was piperacillin/tazobactum and azithromax intravenous. Jan further interviewed the patient to evaluate his exposure to potential infections and he explained that his friend was recently ill with the flu and he had been visiting him frequently in the hospital.

Jan provided detailed information to his family regarding visitation and advised that all visitors must wash their hands upon entering the room and further discussed signs that show how to appropriately wash or use an alcohol gel. She further explained to the patient his rights and advised him to ask all persons providing care to him to assure that they washed their hands prior to touching him and if he has not seen them wash when they approach his bedside to ask the provider to do so (The Joint Commission [TJC], 2005).

NW becomes increasingly ill and requires intubation. Jan sent his bronchial washings for culture. Jan decided to place a right-sided subclavian central venous catheter using maximum barrier precautions.

6.2. ESSENTIAL CONTENT FOR INFECTION CONTROL

Based on the hospital's electronic medical record (EMR), she noted that the patient had been previously evaluated for methicillin resistant staphylococcus aureus (MRSA) and was negative; therefore he did not need to be isolated.

In the United States, the Centers for Disease Control and Prevention (CDC, 2011) has reported that hospitalized patients annually acquire nearly 2 million infections. Many of these hospital acquired infections (HAI) are pan resistant and life-threatening. The use of good hand hygiene compliance by healthcare providers (HCPs) is one of the most important behaviors to prevent the spread of infection. HCPs should practice good hand hygiene practices while providing patient care to decrease the transmission of bloodborne pathogens that may infect a patient. The principles of good hand hygiene include: before patient contact; after contact with blood, body fluids, or contaminated surfaces (even if gloves are worn); before invasive procedures; and after remov-

TABLE 6.1. Area of Aerobic Bacterial Counts on the Skin*.

Body Area/Part	Range/Bacterial Count
Scalp	1×10^6 colony forming unit (CFUs)/cm^2
Axilla	5×10^5 CFUs/cm^2
Abdomen	4×10^4 CFUs/cm^2
Forearm	1×10^4 CFUs/cm^2
Hands	3.9×10^4 to 4.6×10^6 CFU/cm^2

ing gloves (wearing gloves is not enough to prevent the transmission of pathogens in healthcare settings). Since normal human skin is colonized with bacteria on different areas of the body, it is important that healthcare providers are knowledgeable about the varying aerobic bacterial counts found on the skin (Table 6.1).

6.3. HOSPITAL ACQUIRED INFECTIONS IN CRITICAL CARE

Jan was concerned that NW was at risk for a significant septic episode and needed to provide appropriate broad spectrum antibiotics without placing him at risk for further renal failure. Based upon the ICU's antibiogram the medication of choice was piperacillin/tazobactum and azithromax intravenous. Jan further interviewed the patient to evaluate his exposure to potential infections and he explained that his friend was recently ill with the flu and he had been visiting him frequently in the hospital.

NW became increasingly ill and required intubation. Jan sent his bronchial washings for culture. He further needed a central venous catheter access to manage his medications. Jan decided to place a right-sided subclavian central venous catheter using maximum barrier precautions.

He further needed a central venous catheter access to manage his medications.

HAIs are among the most common adverse events occurring during hospital admissions. In 2002, 1.7 million patients suffered from HAIs with an associated 155,668 fatalities, or nearly 10% of the associated population with the highest infection rates in the ICUs (13%) (Klevens *et al.*, 2002). The decision to place a subclavian central venous catheter at the site of insertion is based on data attained from the Institute of Healthcare Improvement (IHI), which demonstrates that catheters placed in the subclavian site have lower infection rates than internal jugular or femoral catheters (IHI.org, 2011). One way to further decrease the likelihood of central line infections is to apply maximal barrier precautions in preparation for line insertion. This is an integral part of the IHI Central Line Bundle and has been correlated with reduction in the rate of central line infection (IHI.org, 2011).

According to the Deshpande study, whenever possible the femoral site should be avoided and the subclavian line site should be preferred over the jugular and femoral sites for non-tunneled catheters in adult patients (Deshpande, Hatem, Ulrich, 2005). For the operator placing the central line and for those assisting in the procedure, maximum barrier precautions mean strict compliance with hand hygiene, wearing a cap, mask, sterile gown and gloves. The cap should cover all hair and the mask should cover the nose and mouth tightly. These precautions are the same as for any other surgical procedure that carries a risk of infection. For the patient, maximal barrier precautions mean covering the patient from head to toe with a sterile drape with a small opening for the site of insertion.

Maximum barrier precautions clearly decrease the odds of developing catheter-related bloodstream infections. Two studies have shown that the odds of developing a central line infection were higher if maximum barrier precautions were not used. For pulmonary artery catheters, the odds ratio of developing infection was more than two times greater for placement without maximum barrier precautions (Mermel *et al.*, 1991; IHI, 2011). A study of similar design found that this rate was six times higher for placement of central line catheters (Raad *et al.*, 1994; IHI, 2011). Therefore, when healthcare providers adhere to a standardized infection prevention protocol during catheter placement the rate of HAIs has been reduced.

6.4. ATTRIBUTABLE COST OF HOSPITAL ACQUIRED INFECTIONS

Upon admission to the ICU, Jan, the acute care nurse practitioner (ACNP), reviewed the laboratory data and completed a thorough review of the patient. Based on the hospital's electronic medical record (EMR), she noted that the patient had been previously evaluated for methicillin resistant staphylococcus aureus (MRSA) and was negative; therefore, he did not need to be isolated.

The attributable cost of HAIs vary depending on the type of infection, and has been estimated to be $34,670 for each surgical site infection and $29,156 for each central line-associated bloodstream infection (CLABSI) (Roberts *et al.*, 2009). Furthermore, the length of hospital stay has been reported to be an average of 9.6 days among patients who develop HAIs (Roberts *et al.*, 2010). CLABSIs constitute one of the most frequent hospital acquired infections in the USA with an associated mortality of up to 25% (CDC, MMWR, 2002). A recent report by the Centers for Disease Control and Prevention showed that in 2009, the number of CLABSIs in American inpatient settings totaled 41,000 events (Vital Signs, 2009).

Interventions aimed at improving compliance with optimal insertion techniques have been proven to decrease the CLABSI rates by as much as 70% (Pronovost *et al.*, 2006). Additionally, maintenance interventions to reduce the bacterial load on patients has proven to be effective at preventing subsequent CLABSIs (Bleasdale *et al.*, 2007). Bacterial skin counts become increasingly important as the ICU patient remains in a hospital setting. The actual bathing and skin cleansing now carries a higher priority. Bleasdale *et al.* (2007), in a 52-week, 2-arm crossover (i.e., concurrent control group) clinical trial study designed with intention-to-treat analysis, determined that when patients bathed daily with chlorhexidine gluconate (CHG) they had a lower incidence of primary bloodstream infections (BSIs) compared with patients who bathed with soap and water.

A recent study was completed to evaluate the effectiveness of different patient hygiene measures to control the incidence of HAIs. The study was completed at a 22-bed medical intensive care unit (MICU) at the John H. Stroger Jr. (Cook County) Hospital, a 464-bed public teaching hospital in Chicago, Illinois. The study population comprised 836 MICU patients. During the first of two study periods (28 weeks), 1 hospital unit was randomly selected to serve as the intervention unit in which patients were bathed daily with 2% CHG-impregnated washcloths (Sage 2% CHG cloths; Sage Products Inc., Cary, Illinois); patients in the concurrent control unit were bathed daily with soap and water. After a 2-week wash-out period at the end of the first period, cleansing methods were crossed over for 24 more weeks. The main outcome measures included the incidences of primary BSIs and clinical (culture-negative) sepsis (primary outcomes) and incidences of other infections (secondary outcomes).

The results demonstrated that patients in the CHG intervention arm were significantly less likely to acquire a primary BSI (4.1 vs. 10.4

infections per 1000 patient days; incidence difference, 6.3 [95% confidence interval, 1.2–11.0]). The incidences of other infections, including clinical sepsis, were similar between the units. Protection against primary BSI by CHG cleansing was apparent after 5 or more days in the MICU. The clinical outcomes associated with this study demonstrated that when protocols are implemented to adhere to a standardized method of patient hygiene, then the rate of HAIs could be decreased.

Although his white blood cell count (WBC) was 2.4 mm^3, his temperature of 35.6 centigrade was concerning.

6.5. HOW TO EFFECTIVELY PROCESS CHANGE

A series of stepwise interventions was implemented at the hospital that admitted NW. The hospital was a 1,500 bed public teaching hospital affiliated with a university setting. The surgical intensive care unit consisted of 40 beds—two adjacent 20-bed units (SICU-A and -B). These two units shared nursing and ancillary staff, and were managed by the same nursing and medical administration. In general, patients colonized with multidrug resistant organisms tended to be allocated in SICU-B and the "clean" patients were allocated in SICU-A. This SICU had 60% transplant patients encompassing liver, kidney, multivisceral, heart, lung, pancreas, and small bowel transplant. The rest of the population encompassed postoperative surgical patients from all subspecialties, including trauma overflow patients. Approximately 10 beds were dedicated to cardiothoracic and cardiovascular patients.

The healthcare team providing care to NW was multidisciplinary. The general surgery patients were managed by a trauma critical care surgeon, fellows, residents, interns, nurse practitioners, registered nurses, patient care technicians, and are followed diligently by an infection control practitioner. The cardiac patients were managed by an anesthesia critical care attending, fellows, residents, nurse practitioners, registered nurses, patient care technicians and are also followed by an infection control practitioner. The management of this was overseen by a director of patient care services for perioperative division. Because of a multidisciplinary effort, the principles of infection control were consistently adhered to within and among all healthcare disciplines. The infection control practitioner provided the structure to communicate issues associated with the signs and symptoms of infection, and prevention strategies were adapted by all healthcare practitioners. Additionally, the infection control practitioner assured that the quality and safety of the patient is the first line of defense against major healthcare associated infections. Therefore, the following quality review study was completed to provide data for all multidisciplinary healthcare providers to prevent Central Line Associated Blood Stream Infections (CLABSIs).

6.5.1. Data Collection Methods for CLABSIs.

CLABSI cases were identified from infection control databases and based on the Centers for Disease and Control's and the National Healthcare Safety Network's definitions. Data were used from the period of time from July 2008 to October 2010. The Infection Control Department kept hard copies of all pertinent medical records reviewed on all positive blood cultures, including the reason for categorizing a positive blood culture as primary versus secondary bacteremia. During this period, only two infection preventionists were in charge of performing CLABSI surveillances in SICU. All cultures were reviewed every shift by nurse practitioners and discussed daily with the infection preventionists. Based upon the discussion of the cultures, the team made decisions to cohort patients. By the end of 2010, all surveillance forms of both primary and secondary bacteremias were retrospectively reviewed and re-categorized accordingly by the Medical Director of Infection Control.

6.5.1.1. Baseline (Phase 1)

CLABSI rates were revised from July 2008 to January 2009. No interventions were performed during this phase; thus these rates were considered as baseline.

6.5.1.2. Scrub the Hub (Phase 2)

This intervention started in SICU-B on February, 2009 and a month later in SICU-A. Scrub the Hub consisted of a 15 second scrub of the intravenous hubs prior to any access using Chloraprep single swabsitck (2% chlorhexidine gluconate and 70% isopropyl alcohol, CareFusion, TX).

6.5.1.3. Education Campaigns

Education campaigns were provided initially to both nurse educators and selected nursing staff ("train-the-trainer"). At the end of the education campaign, over 100 SICU staff nurses were educated by associate nurse managers, nurse educators, or nurse practitioners. Additionally, educational emails regarding technique and rationale for scrub the hub were distributed among the staff. At the beginning of this intervention, the supply manager was in charge of removing all alcohol wipes from patient rooms and nursing stations. Packets of single chlorhexidine swabs were placed next to each patient's bed and in the nursing station. Any procedure requiring alcohol wipes, such as insulin injections, were performed using chlorhexidine swabs. Furthermore, utilization of chlorhexidine swabs was obtained through the hospital's Purchasing Department database dating back to early 2008.

6.5.1.4. Chlorhexidine Wipes (Phase 3)

2% medicated chlorhexidine cloths (Sage®, Cary, IL) replaced soap-and-water baths on August 2009. Staff were trained by nursing educators and Infection Control personnel on the appropriate use of the product. These cloths were used to scrub the body from the neck line to the toes, with special attention not to contact the eyes or ears. Once applied, the product was not rinsed off. All products that were potentially non-compatible with chlorhexidine were removed from the supply area. Cloths were kept warm within the units in warmers provided by the manufacturer. Furthermore, application technique was observed in multiple instances during night shifts (when most baths take place). Utilization data of chlorhexidine cloths were obtained from supply reports.

6.5.1.5. Daily Nursing Rounds (Phase 4)

Starting June 2010, Associate Nurse Managers and Nurse Practitioners conducted daily rounds with each bed side nurse. Daily rounds placed particular attention to an ICU goal list. This list incorporated all safety interventions, including infection control bundles tailored to decrease hospital acquired infections: ventilator associated pneumonia, catheter associated urinary tract infections, and CLABSIs. The Associate Nurse Manager and Nurse Practitioners ensured that any goal not being met was immediately corrected. Additionally, daily nursing sign outs incorporated the ICU goal sheets.

6.5.2. Data Analysis

CLABSI, ventilator associated pneumonias, and catheter associated urinary tract infection rates were calculated monthly (cases in a month ÷ device days ×1000). Intervention groups were grouped into 4 time periods (baseline, scrub the hub, chlorhexidine baths, and nursing rounds), each beginning the month after initiation of the intervention. Data were analyzed by one-way ANOVA with post-hoc Bonferroni comparisons of all groups and post tested for trend over time. Additionally, CLABSI data over the 4 time periods were grouped and analyzed into three groups: Gram-positive cocci, Gram-negative rods, and yeast. CLABSI rates were controlled for rates of ventilator associated pneumonias and catheter associated urinary tract infections. All analyses were performed using PASW Statistics 18.

6.5.3. Results

During the 27 months of data collection, 88 CLABSIs were detected in SICU. The number of CLABSIs ranged from 0 to 8 per month and the average number of monthly device days was 701 (range: 543–873). The mean CLABSI rates went from 7.8 in phase 1 (baseline), to 5.9 in phase 2, 2.8 in phase 3, and 0.4 in phase 4 ($p < 0.0001$). Post-hoc analysis showed differences between phases 1 and 2 ($p < 0.0001$), and 2 and 3 ($p = 0.044$).

CLABSI rates were also analyzed based on the type of organism isolated in blood cultures. Nine cases (10.2%) had two organisms isolated. Gram-positive cocci were the causative organisms in 41 cases: Enterococcus spp. ($n = 23$, 56%), coagulase-negative Staphylococcus spp. ($n = 10$, 24%), and Staphylococcus aureus ($n = 8$, 20%). The CLABSI rates of Gram-positive cocci went from 3.1 in phase 1, to 2.5 in phase 2, 1.6 in phase 3, and 0.7 in phase 4 ($p = .028$). Thirty seven Gram-negative rods were identified: enterics ($n = 19$, 51%), Acinetobacter ($n = 7$, 19%), Pseudomonas ($n = 7$, 19%), and others ($n = 4$, 11%). The rates of CLABSIs caused by Gram-negative organisms went from 3.5 in phase 1, to 2.5 in phase 2, to 0.85 in phase 3, and 0.36 in phase 4 ($p = 0.02$). Similarly, the rate of CLABSIs caused by Candida spp. decreased from 1.9 in phase 1, to 0.92 in phase 2, to 0.29 in phase 3, to zero in phase 4 ($p = 0.029$).

As an aside, monthly rates of ventilator associated pneumonias decreased during the 27 months of observations ($p = 0.008$). However, the only statistically significant decline was detected between phases 1 and 3 ($p = 0.019$). A similar analysis was performed for catheter associated urinary tract infections. No significant differences were noticed over time (0.294). Logistic regression of the CLABSI rates over the

27 months of observation revealed a significant decrease ($R^2 = 0.783$; $p < 0.0001$), even after controlling for rates for ventilator associated pneumonia.

6.5.4. Summary

This process described the importance of implementing infection control strategies for multidisciplinary healthcare professionals in the critical care setting. The use of a detailed sequential implementation of three interventions aimed at decreasing CLABSIs at a single 40-bed SICU were important clinical changes that impacted on patient outcomes. The baseline CLABSI rate was reported to be 7.8 infections per 1,000 device days. After the implementation of scrub-the-hub in February 2009, there was a sudden and persistent decrease in the rate of infection to 5.9. This was followed by the implementation of chlorhexidine baths in August 2009 with a subsequent decrease in infection rates to 2.8. Finally, in June 2010, with the incorporation of daily nursing rounds there was a further decrease in the CLABSI rates to 0.4. Use of these infection prevention procedures demonstrated the need to continue to work as a multidisciplinary healthcare infection control team.

Other interventions that have been successful at decreasing CLABSIs have been categorized into three groups: before, during and post-insertion, as well as the education of the staff to understand the basic principles of IC. Education before insertion included the principles of hand hygiene, avoidance of femoral insertion sites, usage of an all inclusive catheter insertion cart or kit, maximum barrier precautions during catheter insertion, and chlorhexidine skin preparation for catheter insertion. During insertion, education included catheter insertion checklists that reinforced barrier protective techniques. Post-insertion education included disinfection of the port before each access, assessment of the need of catheters during multidisciplinary rounds and removal of all non-essential intravenous and intra-arterial catheters, usage of chlorhexidine for disinfection of the insertion site every 5 to 7 days, placement of chlorhexidine impregnated sponges at the insertion site, and daily chlorhexidine full body baths.

Even though contamination of the intravenous ports are known to be part of the chain of events leading to a bloodstream infection, no previous reports have shown a decrease in the rates of CLABSIs solely by using this intervention. Despite the significant decrease in CLABSI events after the implementation of scrub-the-hub, the unit and facility continue to struggle with attaining a zero rate. Daily chlorhexidine baths were incorporated in the unit as part of a bundle intervention aimed at decreasing the horizontal transmission of multidrug resistant organisms; however, the intervention was instituted across all ICUs at different times, and aimed at decreasing the number of CLABSIs. The SICU's strong nursing and medical leadership were responsible for generating and implementing daily nursing rounds in the SICU. Since the ICU employed a team of critical care nurse practitioners and provided on-going coaching to the nursing staff, daily infection prevention goals were discussed and implemented. The major objective by all HCPs was to practice patient centered care focusing on quality and safe clinical outcomes. The end result was "zero CLABSI" events; thus, a workforce change occurred that incorporated a "culture of safety" within the unit.

Although there were limitations associated with this intervention report, the results demonstrated that when there is increased awareness or adherence by healthcare providers with infection control protocols the rates of CLABSIs were reduced. Although the report is focused on one SICU within the hospital, several of the interventions, such as the use of chlorhexidine baths, were introduced on other hospital units and reduced the rate of HAI rates. Use of the "scrub the hub" protocol was implemented on other units; however, it was less rigorous and not consistent with the daily interventions used in the SICU. Use of daily nursing rounds and SICU infection prevention goal sheets were successfully incorporated only within the SICU. Thus, although limited to one specific area of the hospital (SICU), this report's replication and use on other units was beneficial in reducing the overall rate of HAI in the hospital.

Most likely the use of standardized infection control interventions by the healthcare providers in SICU and strong team leadership decreased CLABSIs to zero. Moreover, the sequential implementation of specific infection control interventions with data that demonstrated the effects of each intervention to the SICU team assisted in the overall success of this program. The "bundle" approach to combating CLABSIs—versus only one intervention—assisted in the elimination of infections.

The use of antibiograms to minimize antibiotic use while providing the most appropriate empiric use of antibiotics until identification and sensitivity was available provided the healthcare team members with data that promoted any overuse of antibiotics. Deescalating broad-spectrum antibiotics as soon as possible facilitates a decrease in the widespread development of pan resistant organisms. Other interventions such as placing patients together with the same and like organisms in non-single room critical care areas may decrease the spread of pan resistant organisms. Additionally the use of surveillance cultures will further facilitate identification of bacterial carriers.

6.6. CONCLUSION AND SUMMARY POINTS

Site Selection
- Subclavian vein (evaluation of patient's clinical condition)
- Internal jugular
- Femoral

Basic Prevention Measures for minimizing all Hospital Acquired Infections

Before Insertion
- Education of all healthcare personnel inserting or handling catheters
- Simulation education
- Nursing driven checklist
- Daily interdisciplinary rounds
- Focused hospital administration on minimizing infection
- Bundled approach
- Following all IHI recommendations

During Insertion
- Checklist with empowerment to halt the procedure if sterile technique is broken
- Hand hygiene
- Use of sterile gloves
- Use of impregnated catheters
- Ultrasound guided insertion (prevention of multiple sticks)
- Maximum barrier protection
- Cleansing of the site with chlorhexidine
- Appropriate site selection
- Applying dressing at end of procedure
- Use of biopatch
- Use of occlusive dressing techniques

Post Insertion Management
- Hand hygiene
- Chlorhexidine baths
- Scrub the hub
- Daily interdisciplinary rounds

- Checklist evaluating need for ongoing catheters use
- Removing multiple catheter sites if no longer needed

Personal Hygiene Measures

- Zero tolerance of non-compliance
- Zero tolerance of HAI

6.7. REFERENCES

Bleasdale, S.C., Trick, W.E., Gonzalez, I.M., *et al.* (2007). Effectiveness of chlorhexi-dine bathing to reduce catheter-associated bloodstream infections in medical inten-sive care unit patients. *Arch. Intern. Med., 22*:167(19):2073–9.

Centers for Disease Control and Prevention. (2011) Vital signs: central line associated blood stream infections, United States, 2001, 2008, and 2009. *MMWR, 60*:243–48.

Centers for Disease Control and Prevention. (2011). Hand Hygiene in Healthcare Set-tings. Retrieved from http://www.cdc.gov/handhygiene/Basics.html

Centers for Disease Control and Prevention (2002). Guideline for Hand Hygiene in Healthcare Settings. Retrieved from http://www.cdc.gov/mmwr/PDF/rr/rr5116.pdf October 25, 2002 / Vol. 51 / No. RR-16

Centers for Disease Control and Prevention. (2002) Guidelines for the Prevention of Intravascular Catheter-Related Infections. *MMWR, 51*:1–29.

Centers for Disease Control and Prevention. (2010) Central Line Associated Blood-stream Infection (CLABSI) Events. Device Associated Module, June 2010. http://www.cdc.gov/nhsn/pdfs/pscmanual/4psc_clabscurrent.pdf

Deshpande, K.S., Hatem, C., Ulrich, H.L., *et al.* (2005) The incidence of infectious complications of central venous catheters at the subclavian, internal jugular, and femoral sites in an intensive care unit population. *Critical Care Medicine, 33*:13.

Institute for Healthcare Improvement (2011). IHI Central Line Bundle: Maximal Bar-rier Precautions Upon Insertion. http://www.ihi.org/knowledge/Pages/Changes/MaximalBarrierPrecautionsUponinsertion.aspx

Klevens, R.M., Edwards, J.R., Richards, C.L. Jr., *et al.* (2002) Estimating health care-associated infections and deaths in U.S. hospitals, 2002. *Public Health Rep., 122*:160–6.

Marschall, J., Mermel, L.A., Classen, D., *et al.* (2008) Strategies to prevent central line-associated bloodstream infections in acute care hospitals. *Infect. Control. Hosp. Epidemiol. 29*(Suppl 1): S22–30.

Mermel, L.A., McCormick, R.D., Springman, S.R. and Maki, D.G. (1991) The patho-genesis and epidemiology of catheter-related infection with pulmonary artery Swan-Ganz catheters: A prospective study utilizing molecular subtyping. *American Jour-nal of Medicine 91*(3B):197S–205S.

Pronovost, P., Needham, D., Berenholtz, S., *et al.* (2006) An intervention to decrease catheter related bloodstream infections in the ICU. *N. Engl. J. Med., 355*:2725–32.

Raad, I.I., Hohn, D.C., Gilbreath, B.J., *et al.* (1994) Prevention of central venous cath-eter-related infections by using maximal sterile barrier precautions during insertion. *Infection Control and Hospital Epidemiology, 15*(4 Pt. 1): 231–238.

Roberts, R.R., Hota, B., Ahmad, I., *et al.* (2009) Hospital and societal costs of antimi-crobial-resistant infections in a Chicago teaching hospital: implications for antibi-otic stewardship. *Clinical Infectious Disease 49*:1175–84.

Roberts, R.R., Scott, R.D. 2nd, Hota, B., *et al.* (2010) Costs attributable to healthcare-acquired infection in hospitalized adults and a comparison of economic methods. *Med. Care 48*:1026–35.

Safdar, N. and Maki, D.G. (2004) The pathogenesis of catheter-related bloodstream infection with noncuffed short-term central venous catheters. *Intensive Care Med., 30*(1): 62-7. Epub 2003 Nov 26.

Scott, R.D. (2009) The Direct Medical costs of Healthcare-Associated Infections in U.S. Hospitals and the Benefits of Prevention. Division of Healthcare Quality Promotion National Center for Preparedness, Detection, and Control of Infectious Diseases Coordinating Center for Infectious Diseases Centers for Disease Control and Prevention. http://www.cdc.gov/ncidod/dhqp/pdf/Scott_CostPaper.pdf

The Joint Commission (2005). Facts about Speak Up Initiatives. Retrieved from www.jointcommission.org/facts_about_speak_up_initiatives

CHAPTER 7

Infection Control in the Emergency Department Settings

MICHELLE WRIGHT MS, RN

A realistic case study of a typical patient who presents to the emergency room in which healthcare personnel do not suspect a contagious or infectious disease. Discussion will include the screening, diagnosis, and tracking of patients who may be at risk for transmitting an infection to other patients or healthcare providers while admitted to the emergency department. Topics will include possible contamination to unknown viruses, bacteria, or biochemical agents.

7.1. CASE PRESENTATION

Lynn is a nurse in a busy urban emergency department (ED). When she arrives at the hospital for her 12-hour shift she notices multiple ambulances in the bay and a full parking lot, she knows it's going to be another busy day. The hospital has been basically full for about 2 weeks; it was January and smack in the middle of flu season. Today was nothing new. Lynn checks in and has been assigned to triage for the day. She sees a wide variety of patients and has to continuously check on the waiting room, where there are around 30 patients waiting to be seen by a physician. Lynn starts standard protocols as needed, and requests all patients with fevers and a cough to wear a surgical mask. She also makes sure that everyone in the waiting room is aware of the hand sanitizing stations and had housekeeping refill empty stations.

To Lynn's dismay, Sam Patel comes in to triage on this busy day to be seen. Sam is a patient Lynn is familiar with; he has been battling cancer on and off over the past 5 years. Seeing him there, she assumes he must no longer be in remission. When she calls Sam to be triaged, he confirms her fears. He just found out he had lung cancer about 3 months ago and was currently undergoing chemotherapy and radiation. He tells Lynn that he coughed up some blood yesterday and the amount seems to be increasing today. He's worried because he has never had this before, and he didn't think it was a normal side effect to his therapy. He had called his oncologist earlier, who told him to go to the ED. Sam said he otherwise felt good, considering his current situation. His vital signs are all within normal limits and he looks remarkably well, considering current cancer therapy. Lynn performs an electrocardiogram, starts a peripheral intravenous line and draws a complete blood count, basic metabolic panel, prothrombin time and partial thromboplastin time to send to the lab and orders a chest radiograph, per standing protocol. Lynn offers Sam a surgical mask, and she tells him it's mostly for his own protection from influenza patients. She sends him back to the waiting room and tells him to listen for an X-ray technician to call him to have a chest x-ray done. Lynn continues on with her day.

In the meantime, Sam is called for his x-ray then goes back to the waiting room. After he has been waiting for 6 hours to be seen, he ask Lynn if she knows how much longer it will be because if he's allowed he would like to get something to eat. Lynn looks to see what his lab and x-ray result indicated. She tells him there are about 5 people still ahead of him. She tells him to wait on eating until she consults with one of the physicians to make sure it's ok first. While Lynn goes to find a physician, Sam finds a drinking fountain and drinks some water. Lynn finds Dr. Wilson and explains Sam case to her. She also tells her his white blood cell count is low, as well as his hemoglobin and hematocrit. She also notices an infiltrate on his chest x-ray that she thought a physician should see. Dr. Wilson pulls up Sam's chart and determines that he would like to see him sooner than later and to send him back next. Lynn returns to the waiting room and calls Sam to tell him the news.

Sam is taken back about an hour later into a regular ED room with a curtain and no door. He dresses in his gown and the nurse and physician assess him. His vitals remain within normal limits. His history includes recent weight loss and fatigue. He said he went back to India about 3 months ago for a wedding. He said he found out the cancer was back about a week before he was supposed to leave and he didn't want to cancel his trip, so he went and started his treatment when he got back from his 2-week stay. Dr. Wilson asks Sam if anyone he was visiting was ill. He said not that he knew of, but he said he did spend quite a bit of time traveling around and he had contact with many people while he was there because of the wedding. He said he would have his wife ask family members if anyone has had any respiratory illnesses around the time of the wedding. Dr. Wilson explains to Sam that they really aren't sure what the infiltrate in the chest x-ray is, that it could be an infection, blood, or fluid related to the cancer, and that the radiologist had recommended a computed tomography (CT) scan to get a better picture. She also told Sam that she wanted to send off some blood cultures and a sputum sample in case it was pneumonia. She was concerned that some of the symptoms of infection may be altered due to his cancer treatment, and she told him his body might not be waging the type of response one would expect.

Sam produces a sputum sample and has his chest CT. However, the results from the CT scan were inconclusive, and sputum sample and blood cultures will take a minimum of 24 hours to produce a meaningful result. Dr. Wilson consults with the oncologist and infectious disease specialists on call and they decide to administer a tuberculin skin test as well, although the test is usually inaccurate in patients receiving immunosuppressive therapy. It has now been 12 hours since Sam sought treatment and it is unclear why he is coughing up blood. The plan is to admit him for further testing and possibly a biopsy of the infiltrate to determine the cause. However, there are no beds available in the hospital, so Sam will have to stay in the ED until one is available. He is moved to a temporary observation area where patients are separated by curtains.

The next day, Lynn is returning to work and gets her assignment and she is shocked to see that Sam will be on her team and that he is in an isolation room. When she gets a report on the patient, she finds out he was just moved to the isolation room an hour ago because he found out one of his relatives that he spent considerable time with at the wedding was hospitalized with TB a week ago. The nurse reporting to Lynn says everyone is nervous because Sam had been ambulatory in the holding area, sharing the bathroom facilities with other patients, and had gone to the cafeteria earlier to have breakfast with his wife. The night nurse told Lynn the previous nurse never told her it was even a consideration that Sam could have an infection. His admitting diagnosis was cancer with lung infiltrate, and since they were short-staffed, she never had time to thoroughly go through the chart. Lynn then goes through the chart to make sure nothing else was overlooked. She also finds that the skin test was never administered, the air exchange had not been activated for Sam's isolation room, and there were no N-95 respirators available. Lynn calls pharmacy to have them prepare the anti-tuberculosis medications ordered with the isolation, collects the proper supplies, dons PPE and enters Sam's room to do an assessment and administer the TB skin test. Sam greets her and asks what the silly mask is for. She explains the situation to Sam and he tells her he thought he just was moved to the room because it was going to be his "room" for the rest of the stay. No one had been in since he was moved to tell him anything. While she administered the test, an isolation room was assigned to him on a medical surgical unit.

7.2. ESSENTIAL CONTENT FOR INFECTION CONTROL SKILLS

Identification and management of patients with infectious diseases should begin immediately upon entry to the Emergency Department (ED) to best protect patients and staff from the spread of infection. The increasing varieties of healthcare-associated infections (HAIs) are alarming, but other infectious disease can also spread rapidly through an ED—such as severe acute respiratory syndrome (SARS)—and are not normally associated with healthcare-associated acquisition. Unidentified case patients are the greatest source of transmission for highly contagious disease. Therefore, prompt assessment of patients presenting with symptoms of highly infectious disease is warranted. Suspicions should be raised when patients have recently traveled abroad, have frequent contact with healthcare facilities, or had contact with confirmed cases of contagious disease. Chen and colleagues (2005) analyzed the spread of SARS and determined that the sooner EDs implemented strict infection control measures when a SARS outbreak was identified impacted how many employees became ill. Hospitals that implemented procedures quickly reported only 9% of employees staying home for fever, while 47% called in for fever in areas that delayed implementation of strict protocols. When patients present to the ED with potentially devastating infectious agents, it is imperative that the infection control personnel and administrators be notified to initiate the proper protocols. Confirmation of infectious disease may not occur in the ED; however, steps can be initiated to prevent the spread of disease.

7.3. PRECAUTIONS

Lynn starts standard protocols as needed, and requests all patients with fevers and a cough to wear a surgical mask. She also makes sure that everyone in the waiting room is aware of the hand sanitizing stations and had housekeeping refill empty stations.

Healthcare providers in all settings should practice standard precautions. ED staff must be particularly attuned to symptoms of disease that may be infectious in nature because the ED is where most patients present to the hospital with health concerns. Practitioners responsible for triage must have exceptional assessment skills and should readily apply masks to patients presenting with a cough and remind patients of the importance of good hand hygiene. The locations of hand sanitizers and sinks should be pointed out to patients and they should also be reminded to cough into their sleeves or tissue to prevent the spread of infection to other patients awaiting treatment (Harding, Almquist and Hashemi, 2011). To help remind patients, and insure information reaches patients even prior to triage assessment, placement of "Cover Your Cough" posters can be placed where patients enter the waiting room, triage area, treatment areas, and in restrooms. The flyers are also available for download in multiple languages on the CDC website. Patients that present to the ED should have the appropriate transmission based precautions initiated immediately; particularly if the patient's recent history indicates the symptoms may be infectious in nature. Other healthcare providers should be notified of suspected infections to ensure infection prevention measures are followed when care transitions from one provider to another.

7.4. UNKNOWN ILLNESS

He tells Lynn that he coughed up some blood yesterday and the amount seems to be increasing today. He's worried because he has never had this before, and he didn't think it was a normal side effect to his therapy. He called his oncologist earlier, who told him to go to the ED. Sam said he otherwise felt good, for his current situation. His vital signs are all within normal limits and he looks remarkably well considering current cancer therapy.

7.4.1. Respiratory

Respiratory illnesses have the potential to spread quickly and patients frequently seek treatment in the ED for respiratory issues. Most respiratory pathogens that cause illness, like influenza, are spread by droplets produced by coughing and sneezing and do not require special ventilation. Rooming such a patient in a negative pressure isolation room is unnecessary since droplets can only travel 1–2 meters. However, the use of surgical masks and isolating the patient to a private room can help contain the pathogen to the infected host. Occasionally, a higher level of precaution may be warranted when pandemics of highly lethal pathogens spread by droplets occur, such as SARS (Puro et al., 2008). Since ED employees have very high risk of exposure to respiratory infections, vaccinations should be encouraged for providers when available.

Additionally, some respiratory pathogens are airborne, such as tuberculosis (TB), and require the use of a respirator mask and negative pressure rooms to prevent the spread of disease to healthcare providers and other patients. Infections caused by SARS, H1N1, and multidrug resistant TB may result in death and can spread quickly when in an overcrowded ED. Strains of completely drug resistant TB have been identified in Mumbai in December of 2011, and without proper infection control measures, these infections could become widespread (Udwadia et al., 2011). Ideally, all patients presenting to the ED with respiratory symptoms should wear a surgical mask to help protect other patients and staff, since it is difficult to diagnosis a specific ailment without cultures. When patients present to the ED with a fever and respiratory symptoms, staff providing care for them may also don surgical masks to protect themselves from infection. Wearing a surgical mask as well as N95 respirators will prevent providers from acquiring many common infectious respiratory ailments, such as influenza (Loeb et al., 2009). Patients presenting with fever and cough are more likely to have a flu virus like H1N1 during a pandemic than those who do not; however, children and immunocompromised patients may present with atypical symptoms (Lee et al., 2011). ED providers should remain cognizant of patterns of respiratory illness in the area they live, as well as general trends since travel between cities, states, and countries is much more common that it was decades ago.

Further compounding the issue is the human immunodeficiency virus (HIV), because it increases susceptibility to infections like TB. Certain populations, such as the homeless, are at a higher risk of acquiring these infections and tend to utilize the ED as a method of primary care.

Further, there are higher rates of TB infection in ED staff (Behrman and Shofer, 1998; Escombe *et al.*, 2010; Jiamjarasrangsi *et al.*, 2005). This could be because they are more likely than other healthcare staff to be exposed to unidentified cases and to interact closely with infected patients without taking necessary precautions. Additionally, TB may not be diagnosed until well after a patient has been admitted. There have also been a number of outbreaks of TB in EDs in areas with traditionally low incidence of TB. Furthermore, patients with TB tend to make multiple ED visits prior to diagnosis with the disease, increasing staff risk of acquiring the disease due to multiple exposures (Long *et al.*, 2002; Sokolove *et al.*, 1994). ED practitioners can use decision tools to better target patients that may have TB. All ED providers should know seven criteria that have been associated with TB: apical infiltrate, weight loss, history of TB, immigrants, cavitation, homeless, and history of incarceration (Moran *et al.*, 2009). If patients do not have any of the criteria, it is unlikely the presenting patient has TB. Clinical decision tools should be utilized to correctly appropriate patients to limited isolation rooms.

7.4.2. Bloodborne Infections

Providers in the ED are frequently exposed to blood and blood products. It is imperative that gloves be worn anytime there is potential contact with blood, including drawing blood samples and giving injections. Providers are also exposed to sharps more frequently than some other settings since invasive procedures frequently occur in the ED, including but not limited to: blood draws and intravenous line insertion, central line placement, suturing, and emergency surgical procedures (i.e., thoracotomy, etc.). Furthermore, providers may be exposed to patients actively bleeding from lacerations, burns, gunshot wounds, and traumatic amputations. Care should be taken by all providers to wear the appropriate personal protective equipment (PPE) when patients present with active bleeding.

Since sharps injuries do occur in the ED, there has been some debate if providers and patients need to be tested prior to receiving care in the setting for various bloodborne pathogens. The American College of Emergency Physicians (ACEP) (2011) does not recommend mandatory hepatitis or HIV testing in order for patients to receive care in emergency settings; however, they do encourage universal HIV screening. The CDC is also reviewing screening guidelines for hepatitis C, and may encourage screening for all persons born between 1945 and 1965 in the near future.

At the very least, patients seeking treatment in the ED for blood or body fluid exposure, sexual assault, and sexually transmitted infections should be tested for HIV (Merchant and Catanzaro, 2009). Most healthcare facilities require staff to obtain hepatitis B vaccination prior to working. However, exemptions can be claimed for religious or other reasons at some organizations. Additionally, HIV seropositive employees should not be restricted from providing emergency care unless the disease state hinders their ability to perform required duties (ACEP, 2011).

Patients should be assessed for recent international travel when presenting to the ED, since they could be infected with a number of agents not endemic to the United States. Additionally, incidence of certain bloodborne disease is much higher in other countries, such as HIV, and risk behaviors and potential exposure to blood or body fluids while traveling should specifically be assessed. All vaccines and travel medicine the patient has been taking should also be carefully investigated. Patients presenting with a fever that have recently traveled to areas such as Sub-Saharan Africa and Southeast Asia may require blood cultures, malaria smear, nasal swabs for influenza, hepatitis and HIV testing. It is not uncommon for patients traveling from these areas to present with more than one illness. Patients who acquire dangerous bloodborne illness while traveling, as well as the public, will benefit from early identification and treatment of the illnesses (Siikamäki *et al.*, 2011).

7.4.3. Diarrheal Disease

In addition to respiratory ailments, patients frequently seek treatment in the ED for gastrointestinal complaints. Practitioners should be aware that many pathogenic agents that cause infectious diarrhea are highly contagious. Strict adherence to hand hygiene is paramount in preventing the spread of infection when caring for patients with diarrheal illness. Norovirus is the most frequent cause of gastroenteritis in the United States, and patients suspected of having the illness should be placed on contact isolation to help prevent the spread of the disease. Healthcare workers that become ill should not be allowed to return to work until at least 2 days after symptoms have resolved—at which time they should not longer be able to spread the infection. Additionally, rotavirus is the most common cause of gastroenteritis in children, and the same precautions should be followed as for norovirus. Oral vaccines for rotavirus are available and recommended by the CDC. ED providers can educate parents that a vaccine is available and the parents may wish to consider vaccinating other children in the household.

Campylobacter is associated with traveler's diarrhea and is the most common cause of bacterial diarrhea worldwide. *Salmonella* and *Clostridium difficile* are other bacterial agents that cause severe diarrheal illness and may quickly spread and contaminate the ED environment. *C. difficile* is the most problematic of the three agents because the bacteria produces spores that are not killed by alcohol-based hand sanitizers that have become commonplace. Additionally, the spores can live on surfaces and inanimate objects for weeks, and become active if acquired by a vulnerable individual. Further, the spores are not killed by traditional cleaners used in most EDs and require the use of bleach solution for proper disinfection. Therefore, it is important that all healthcare providers use only soap and water for hand hygiene and appropriate bleach products for environmental disinfection for patients suspected of having *C. difficile*. Additionally, these patients should be placed on contact isolation and ideally have their own private commode or bathroom. *Camplyobacter* and *Salmonella* infections are usually self-limiting and only require oral rehydration therapy. Antibiotics may be of some benefit if given early during the course of illness. Patients infected with *C. difficile* will likely require antibiotic treatment to resolve the infection. Patients presenting with diarrheal illness may also be screened for *Escherichi coli* pathotypes (Nataro *et al.*, 2006) or for parasites based on recent travel and medical history.

7.5. BIOCHEMICAL AGENTS

In the event of a biochemical agent being used as a weapon, it is likely the affected will be brought to an ED for treatment. EDs should have a plan in place to contain and treat patients that may present with anthrax, radioactive materials, SARS, monkeypox, or other dangerous and highly contagious agents. Facilities should also have a disaster management plan in place and it is the staff's duty to be familiar with such plans. Some facilities may transform an existing unit, like an oncology unit, into an isolation ward, whereas others may have a temporary biocontainment unit that will be constructed in the event of an attack or outbreak of a highly infectious agent. In order for staff to be familiar with the policies and equipment, practice drills should be routinely performed. At the University of Nebraska Medical Center, practice drills are completed quarterly and performance is evaluated upon drill completion to address areas that need improvement (Beam *et al.*, 2010). Performing regular drills will help prevent issues that occurred during a recent SARS outbreak. When the outbreak occurred, a number of healthcare providers in Canada became ill after breaching infection control policies because many were unaware of how to properly don and doff personal protective equipment (Ofner-Agostini *et al.*, 2006).

Patients suspected of being exposed to biochemical agents should be quickly triaged for life threatening complication and decontaminated prior to entry into the ED, whenever possible (Vinson, 2007). Many hospitals have decontamination areas in ambulance bays or near a separate entrance that leads directly to isolation rooms. A hot zone, contaminated area, and cold zone (clean area), should be established and clearly demarcated for any patient that has been exposed to a biochemical threat. After a patient has been decontaminated, they should be quarantined in a designated cold zone that is separate from other patients. After the patient has been decontaminated, they should be reassessed for wounds and other medical problems needing treatment. If a patient presents directly to triage area after exposure to a biochemical hazard, they should immediately be taken to a decontamination room. The provider must carefully consider the route to the decontamination room to limit hazard exposure to others. Any area the patient may have contaminated upon approach to the triage area should be quarantined and decontaminated. Anyone who came in contact with the patient should also be decontaminated and placed in isolation. In the event that a large number of people are exposed to a biochemical threat, separate buildings many be designated for decontamination, isolation, and treatment of exposed individuals. This strategy has been successfully applied during the SARS outbreak to help limit the spread of infection (McDonald *et al.*, 2004).

7.6. TRAUMA

Trauma patients pose unique challenges to emergency personnel because many of the patients cannot speak or are disoriented and unable to give information about their previous medical history. Trauma patients may have profuse bleeding or cerebrospinal fluid drainage that could be infectious. Strict universal precautions should be maintained when caring for such patients. Additionally, care should be taken to properly clean and disinfect all reusable trauma equipment after use. Lee, Levy, and Walker (2006) discovered that 15% of equipment used for stabilizing trauma patients was visibly soiled with blood and, with forensic testing, found an additional 42% of items to be contaminated with blood invisible to the naked eye. Items contaminated with body fluids pose a threat to healthcare worker and patient health, and providers should be aware that objects used to transport trauma patients may be contaminated with potentially infectious materials.

7.7. TRAVEL

He said he went back to India about 3 months ago for a wedding. He said he found out the cancer was back about a week before he was supposed to leave and he didn't want to cancel his trip, so he went and started his treatment when he got back from his 2-week stay.

The increase in international travel over the past few decades increases risk that disease transmission may occur on a global scale. When Siikmaki and colleagues (2011) evaluated common diagnoses of returning travelers, they found that most patients (368/417) were referred to the ED by another physician for further evaluation. Diarrhea, respiratory, and febrile illness accounted for 63% of diagnosed illness and 10% of patients had more than one infection. ED workers should be sure to assess recent travel in patients, particularly when they present with fever, diarrhea, or respiratory illness, and to consider that the patient may be infected with multiple pathogens. Providers should also do their best to stay informed about current outbreaks of infectious diseases and consult with an infectious disease or travel medicine specialist when they are unfamiliar with pathogens endemic to areas the patient traveled to. Facilities may also consider implementing protocols for recent travelers, like those in Finland, particularly if people in the community are known to travel frequently to areas that have known endemic pathogens such as malaria. For example, when people have been to malaria-endemic regions and present with unexplained fever, the following tests are completed:

• Malaria smear
• Two blood cultures
• C reactive protein
• Hemoglobin, white blood cell, & platelet count
• Sodium, potassium, & liver enzymes
• Urine sample
• Chest radiograph

Labs to include in protocols should be diagnostic for the travel related illnesses that may be most likely to occur based on the community the hospital is serving. If there are no regular patterns of travel in the community the ED serves, consulting with a travel medicine or infectious disease specialist could help ensure necessary diagnostic tests are completed.

7.8. EQUIPMENT SHARING

Lynn performs an electrocardiogram . . . Sam is called for his x-ray then goes back to the waiting room . . . Sam finds a drinking fountain and drinks some water.

The spread of infectious disease in the ED via fomites is a particularly challenging issue because quick patient turnover may result in substandard disinfection of objects between patients. It is not uncommon for thermometers, electrocardiogram (ECG) lead wires, IV poles, or medication pumps to be used for multiple patients in rapid succession. Multiple species of *Staphylococcus*, *Acinetobacter*, *Entercoccus*, and *Streptococcus* have been isolated from ECG wires that had been cleaned and ready for reuse in various settings, with the highest contamination rates in EDs (Albert *et al.*, 2010).

Proper cleaning of instruments and equipment between patients can eliminate the spread of infection via fomites. For example, cleaning ultrasound probes with quaternary ammonia germicidal wipes removed methicillin-resistant *Staphylococcus aureus* (MRSA) from 90% of probes, and removed MRSA from all probes if they were partially cleaned prior to using the wipes (Frazee *et al.*, 2011). Materials that were used for patients suspected of having *Clostridium difficile* or norovirus should always be cleaned with bleach to prevent the spread of infection since traditional cleaners are ineffective (Cohen *et al.*, 2010; Weber *et al.*, 2010). Providers should ensure rooms have been properly cleaned between patients, including decontamination of stretchers, guardrails, monitors, reusable wire leads, and intravenous infusion pumps. Equipment used for multiple patients within in the department, such as blood glucose monitoring devices and thermometers, should be cleaned immediately after use.

Furthermore, a large number of EDs still utilize curtains to separate patients or use them for privacy in lieu of doors on rooms. If curtains are being used, there should be a supply of curtains available to change out the curtains after a patient that has been on isolation precautions is discharged or moved to another unit. Changing the curtains is particularly important after a room has been inhabited with a patient infected with pathogens like *C. difficile* that are capable of being infectious for long periods of time on fomites. Often times, it is unclear how often curtains are changed or cleaned. They should be regularly changed or disinfected; it likely is not cost effective or efficient to change them between all patients. However, a regular cleaning schedule should be established and they need to be changed after a patient with an infection requiring transmission-based precautions has stayed in the room.

7.9. PATIENT MOBILITY

. . . everyone is nervous because Sam had been ambulatory in the holding area, sharing the bathroom facilities with other patients, and had gone to the cafeteria earlier to have breakfast with his wife.

Many patients that present to the ED with potentially dangerous infectious disease will be ambulatory. If the team determines that a patient's condition warrants transmission-based precautions it is imperative that the reason for the isolation be explained to the patient and any visitors they have. In the case of biochemical hazard exposure, the patient and anyone they were exposed to may potentially be quarantined together if there are not contraindications. Any patient that has transmission-based precautions should have transport through the hospital kept to an absolute minimum. Tests and procedures should be done at the bedside whenever possible to prevent exposure to others. If transport of the patient is necessary, the receiving staff should be notified of the patient's level of transmission-based precaution and why they have them. The staff should prepare the receiving area accordingly and don the proper PPE. Further, patients with respiratory precautions should be transported wearing a mask. Infected patients should not be transported through main thoroughfares. Some of the current electronic health records have a feature that flags patients that have isolation precautions ordered; it is essential to include what the causative agent is so that all providers will be alerted to the patient's condition. Some facilities also have bed-tracking devices, allowing for easy patient tracking.

7.10. OVERCROWDING

> . . . around 30 patients waiting to be seen by a physician . . .
> she sends him back to the waiting room . . .

EDs frequently have issues with overcrowding. The risk of overcrowding may be higher when there is an infectious disease outbreak because of an increased need for care, and will likely include a large number of uninfected people that are worried they may be. Many hospitals may have relatively few open beds for admitting new patients, even when an outbreak is not occurring. So, when the system is additionally stressed by a large influx of patients, it can create major issues in the ED because there is nowhere for patients to be admitted to. When there are no beds open to admit patients, they end up staying long hours, sometimes days, in the ED and receive routine care there. When this happens, it decreases the ED's ability to see and treat new patients because they have no available space to assess and treat patients. The lack of throughput results in waiting rooms full of very sick patients who are in very close proximity to one another. This scenario creates an optimal environment for disease transmission and is not uncommon in EDs, even when there is not an outbreak. Additionally, the ED may treat patients in hallways or the triage area when regular ED rooms are no longer available. Whenever possible, patients that are suspected of having a highly contagious infectious disease should have priority placement in an isolation room, or cohorted with patients with the same ailment (when known) with a designated staff team so that they don't spread the infection to other patients.

7.11. EMPIRICAL ANTIBIOTIC THERAPY

> Lynn calls pharmacy to have them prepare the anti-tuberculous medications ordered with the isolation.

Antimicrobial therapy is frequently initiated in emergency departments. With the increasing incidence of multi-drug resistant (MDR) organisms, steps should be taken to ensure organizations incorporate EDs into antimicrobial stewardship programs. Frequently, EDs are not incorporated into programs since it is difficult to implement to main tenets of stewardship when patients are rapidly transitioned to other units, acute care facilities, or discharged. Antimicrobial therapy is costly to hospitals and can lead to poor patient outcomes if the chosen therapy is inappropriate. At the very least, the type of medication, route, dose, and duration of therapy should be assessed when blood culture results are completed to improve care and reduce antimicrobial resistance (Dellit *et al.*, 2007). Acquisto and Baker (2011) described two separate stewardship programs that were managed by an emergency pharmacist. The programs allowed for the pharmacist to follow up on blood culture results either with the appropriate physicians or directly with the patient. The pharmacist-run programs seemed to decrease the readmission rates, workload for emergency medicine providers, and decrease the time to follow-up. ED antimicrobial stewardship programs need further development to decrease antimicrobial resistance and inappropriate treatment.

Furthermore, acquisition of infections caused by antibiotic-resistant bacteria in the community is becoming more and more common. For example, extended-spectrum β-lactamase (ESBL)-producing bacteremia is an infection that should be considered for patients presenting with sepsis since it occurs in patients from the community, not only those already admitted to the hospital. A retrospective study analyzing patients seen in the ED that had ESBL were prescribed inappropriate antibiotic therapy in 56 of the 64 identified cases, which also resulted in longer hospital stays (Lin *et al.*, 2011). Risk factors associated with ESBL bacteremia were antibiotic use within 6 months, urinary catheterization, and hospital-acquired infections (Lin *et al.*, 2011). This many not include all predisposing factors, although these are issues that should be assessed when obtaining information from patients prior to the ordering of antibiotics. If a patient presents with any of the risk factors, the provider may wish to consider a carbapenem for treatment of patients with serious bacteremia (Paterson and Bonomo, 2005).

7.12. NOVEL APPROACHES

In the event of a pandemic, EDs will need to be creative in methods to safely treat patients without causing cross contamination. ED's disaster plans may need to be used or modified in these situations to accommodate a large influx of patients. For example, many ED disaster plans have a tent that can be set up to treat patients exposed to a biohazard agent. In the event of a flu pandemic, this temporary treatment area could be set up as an alternate triage or treatment area for patients with the suspected illness. Triaging suspected flu patients in an alternate area would help decrease the risk of infection for patients requiring medical treatment not related to the pandemic infection. Weiss and colleagues (2010) have been working to develop a new way to quickly triage patients in the event of a flu outbreak. They developed a plan for "drive-through" assessment and treatment. They utilized a parking structure as a designated area to screen and treat patients with flu-like symptoms. The study used volunteers who presented to a screening nurse prior to entrance to the ED. Volunteers were given a card with medical information and answers to give the medical personnel in the study. The information was abstracted from de-identified patient data that had previously been treated in the ED. Complete assessments were done by the staff, although they documented the clinical information that was on the volunteer's card. They were able to rapidly assess, diagnose, and treat patients while limiting exposure to patients not presenting with symptoms. Similar approaches will likely be needed in pandemic situations to control the spread of disease.

7.13. SUMMARY POINTS

- Unidentified cases are the greatest source of transmission for highly contagious disease
- Transmission-based precautions should be initiated as soon as possible
- Patients should be told the locations of sinks, hand sanitizer, and masks
- All patients with potential respiratory infections should wear a mask, when possible
- Disaster drills should occur frequently
- Equipment and environment need meticulous cleaning between patients
- Recent travel must be assessed in patients
- Patient transport should be minimized.
- Antimicrobial stewardship should begin in the Emergency Department
- Disaster plans may need to be implemented during pandemics

7.14. REFERENCES

Acquisto, N.M. and Baker, S.N. (2011). Antimicrobial stewardship in the emergency department. *Journal of Pharmacy Practice,* 24(2): 196–202. doi:10.1177/0897190011400555

Albert, N.M., Hancock, K., Murray, T., *et al.* (2010). Cleaned, ready-to-use, reusable electrocardiographic lead wires as a source of pathogenic microorganisms. *American Journal of Critical Care: An Official Publication, American Association of Critical-Care Nurses,* 19(6): e73-80. doi:10.4037/ajcc2010304

American College of Emergency Physicians (ACEP). (2011). Blood-borne infections in emergency medicine. Policy statement. *Annals of Emergency Medicine,* 58(1): 111–112. doi:10.1016/j.annemergmed.2011.04.026

Beam, E.L., Boulter, K.C., Freihaut, F., Schwedhelm, S. and Smith, P.W. (2010). The Nebraska experience in biocontainment patient care. *Public Health Nursing (Boston, Mass.),* 27(2): 140–147. doi:10.1111/j.1525-1446.2010.00837.x

Behrman, A.J. and Shofer, F.S. (1998). Tuberculosis exposure and control in an urban emergency department. *Annals of Emergency Medicine,* 31(3): 370–375.

Chen, W.K., Wu, H.D., Lin, C.C. and Cheng, Y.C. (2005). Emergency department response to SARS, Taiwan. *Emerging Infectious Diseases,* 11(7): 1067–1073.

Cohen, S.H., Gerding, D.N., Johnson, S., *et al.* (2010). Clinical practice guidelines for clostridium difficile infection in adults: 2010 update by the Society for Healthcare Epidemiology of America (SHEA) and the Infectious Diseases Society of America (IDSA). *Infection Control and Hospital Epidemiology: The Official Journal of the Society of Hospital Epidemiologists of America,* 31(5): 431–455. doi:10.1086/651706

Dellit, T.H., Owens, R.C., McGowan, J.E.,Jr., *et al.* (2007). Infectious Diseases Society of America and the Society For Healthcare Epidemiology of America guidelines for developing an institutional program to enhance antimicrobial stewardship. *Clinical Infectious Diseases: An Official Publication of the Infectious Diseases Society of America,* 44(2): 159–177. doi:10.1086/510393

Escombe, A.R., Huaroto, L., Ticona, E., *et al.* (2010). Tuberculosis transmission risk and infection control in a hospital emergency department in Lima, Peru. *The International Journal of Tuberculosis and Lung Disease: The Official Journal of the International Union Against Tuberculosis and Lung Disease,* 14(9): 1120–1126.

Frazee, B.W., Fahimi, J., Lambert, L. and Nagdev, A. (2011). Emergency department ultrasonographic probe contamination and experimental model of probe disinfection. *Annals of Emergency Medicine,* 58(1): 56–63. doi:10.1016/j.annemergmed.2010.12.015

Harding, A.D., Almquist, L.J. and Hashemi, S. (2011). The use and need for standard precautions and transmission-based precautions in the emergency department. *Journal of Emergency Nursing: JEN: Official Publication of the Emergency Department Nurses Association,* 37(4): 367-73; quiz 424–425. doi:10.1016/j.jen.2010.11.017

Jiamjarasrangsi, W., Hirunsuthikul, N. and Kamolratanakul, P. (2005). Tuberculosis among health care workers at King Chulalongkorn Memorial Hospital, 1988–2002. *The International Journal of Tuberculosis and Lung Disease: The Official Journal of the International Union Against Tuberculosis and Lung Disease,* 9(11): 1253–1258.

Lee, J.B., Levy, M. and Walker, A. (2006). Use of a forensic technique to identify blood contamination of emergency department and ambulance trauma equipment. *Emergency Medicine Journal: EMJ,* 23(1): 73–75. doi:10.1136/emj.2005.025346

Lee, T.C., Taggart, L.R., Mater, B., Katz, K. and McGeer, A. (2011). Predictors of pandemic influenza infection in adults presenting to two urban emergency departments, Toronto, 2009. *CJEM,* 13(1): 7–12.

Lin, J.N., Chen, Y.H., Chang, L.L., *et al.* (2011). Clinical characteristics and out-comes of patients with extended-spectrum beta-lactamase-producing bacteremias in the emergency department. *Internal and Emergency Medicine, 6*(6): 547–555. doi:10.1007/s11739-011-0707-3

Loeb, M., Dafoe, N., Mahony, J., *et al.* (2009). Surgical mask vs N95 respirator for preventing influenza among health care workers: A randomized trial. *JAMA: The Journal of the American Medical Association, 302*(17): 1865–1871. doi:10.1001/jama.2009.1466

Long, R., Zielinski, M., Kunimoto, D. and Manfreda, J. (2002). The emergency depart-ment is a determinant point of contact of tuberculosis patients prior to diagnosis. *The International Journal of Tuberculosis and Lung Disease: The Official Journal of the International Union Against Tuberculosis and Lung Disease, 6*(4): 332–339.

McDonald, L.C., Simor, A.E., Su, I.J., *et al.* (2004). SARS in healthcare facilities, To-ronto and Taiwan. *Emerging Infectious Diseases, 10*(5): 777–781.

Merchant, R.C. and Catanzaro, B.M. (2009). HIV testing in US EDs, 1993-2004. *The American Journal of Emergency Medicine, 27*(7): 868–874. doi:10.1016/j.ajem.2008.06.019

Moran, G.J., Barrett, T.W., Mower, W.R., Krishnadasan, A., Abrahamian, F.M., Ong, S. and EMERGEncy ID NET Study Group. (2009). Decision instrument for the isolation of pneumonia patients with suspected pulmonary tuberculosis admitted through US emergency departments. *Annals of Emergency Medicine 53*(5): 625–632. doi:10.1016/j.annemergmed.2008.07.027

Nataro, J.P., Mai, V., Johnson, J., Blackwelder, W.C., Heimer, R., Tirrell, S. and Hir-shon, J.M. (2006). Diarrheagenic escherichia coli infection in Baltimore, Maryland, and New Haven, Connecticut. *Clinical Infectious Diseases: An Official Publication of the Infectious Diseases Society of America, 43*(4): 402–407. doi:10.1086/505867

Ofner-Agostini, M., Gravel, D., McDonald, L.C., *et al.* (2006). Cluster of cases of se-vere acute respiratory syndrome among Toronto healthcare workers after implemen-tation of infection control precautions: A case series. *Infection Control and Hospital Epidemiology: The Official Journal of the Society of Hospital Epidemiologists of America, 27*(5): 473–478. doi:10.1086/504363

Paterson, D.L. and Bonomo, R.A. (2005). Extended-spectrum beta-lactamases: A clinical update. *Clinical Microbiology Reviews, 18*(4): 6570–686. doi:10.1128/CMR.18.4.657-686.2005

Puro, V., Fusco, F.M., Lanini, S., Nisii, C. and Ippolito, G. (2008). Risk management of febrile respiratory illness in emergency departments. *The New Microbiologica 31*(2): 165–173.

Siikamaki, H.M., Kivela, P.S., Sipila, P.N., *et al.* (2011). Fever in travelers return-ing from malaria-endemic areas: Don't look for malaria only. *Journal of Travel Medicine, 18*(4): 239–244. doi:10.1111/j.1708-8305.2011.00532.x; 10.1111/j.1708-8305.2011.00532.x

Sokolove, P.E., Mackey, D., Wiles, J. and Lewis, R.J. (1994). Exposure of emergency department personnel to tuberculosis: PPD testing during an epidemic in the com-munity. *Annals of Emergency Medicine, 24*(3): 418–421.

Udwadia, Z.F., Amale, R.A., Ajbani, K.K. and Rodrigues, C. (2011). Totally drug-resistant tuberculosis in India. *Clinical Infectious Diseases: An Official Publication of the Infectious Diseases Society of America,* doi:10.1093/cid/cir889

Vinson, E. (2007). Managing bioterrorism mass casualties in an emergency depart-ment: Lessons learned from a rural community hospital disaster drill. *Disaster Man-agement & Response: DMR: An Official Publication of the Emergency Nurses As-sociation, 5*(1): 18–21. doi:10.1016/j.dmr.2006.11.003

Weber, D.J., Rutala, W.A., Miller, M.B., Huslage, K. and Sickbert-Bennett, E. (2010). Role of hospital surfaces in the transmission of emerging health care-associated pathogens: Norovirus, clostridium difficile, and acinetobacter species. *American Journal of Infection Control, 38*(5 Suppl 1): S25–33. doi:10.1016/j.ajic.2010.04.196

Weiss, E.A., Ngo, J., Gilbert, G.H. and Quinn, J.V. (2010). Drive-through medicine: A novel proposal for rapid evaluation of patients during an influenza pandemic. *Annals of Emergency Medicine, 55*(3): 268–273. doi:10.1016/j.annemergmed.2009.11.025

CHAPTER 8

Infection Control in Primary Care Settings

CAROL PATTON, PhD., RN, FNP and
DENISE M. KORNIEWICZ PhD., RN, FAAN

This chapter will discuss infection control practices commonly known to occur in primary care settings, clinics and primary care offices. A case study with a simple procedure will be presented and discussion about the preventive aspects of infection control will be reviewed. Topics that will be discussed include excision of a wound, simple suturing techniques, use of cauterization, use of simple instruments and the transmission of infection.

8.1. CASE PRESENTATION

Amy is a certified registered nurse practitioner working in a small, rural primary care clinic that serves minority and under-represented populations. Daily, an average of fifty patients, families, and significant others pass through the waiting room and clinic setting. Amy is concerned about the current methods of cleaning and sterilizing instruments commonly used in patient procedures such as suturing, cauterization, vaginal instruments, and other instruments, since staff seem to have difficulty using standardized protocols for disinfection.

Amy has always been accustomed to working in large tertiary care centers where someone else has had to worry about disinfection or the sterilization of instruments and monitoring infection control practices. Amy is concerned about the lack of any standard procedure for cleansing and sterilizing the simple instruments used in primary care. Additionally, she is worried that the nursing assistants who now care for the instruments and clean the patient rooms may not be knowledgeable about the principles associated with infection control.

129

Today, Amy noticed a nursing assistant rinsing a non-disposable vaginal speculum with water in the sink of the exam room and then returning it to the drawer for use for the next patient. Amy couldn't believe what she had just witnessed and is now concerned that policies about infection control in primary care need to be established to handle simple instruments. She also witnessed a healthcare provider perform an incision and drainage of an abscess on a patient that she suspected to have community-acquired methicillin-resistant Staphylococcus aureus (CA-MRSA) without gloves.

Amy is terrified about spreading infectious diseases from one patient to another—as well as other healthcare providers—in the primary care setting, and wants to help create an infection control and prevention model that focuses on patients and assists healthcare providers (HCPs) in primary care settings to embrace the standards of infection prevention.

8.2. ESSENTIAL CONTENT FOR INFECTION CONTROL SKILLS

Amy is concerned about the current methods of cleaning and sterilizing instruments commonly used in patient procedures such as suturing, cauterization, vaginal instruments and other instruments, since staff seem to have difficulty using standardized protocols for disinfection.

Over the past decade, more and more patients are receiving care in primary care versus tertiary care settings. Patients are seen for follow-up post acute care and for simple procedures performed by primary care providers. An infection control and prevention program in these primary care settings must be embraced by healthcare providers (HCPs) to protect the patient populations which they serve. For example, more and more vulnerable and "at-risk" patients are being cared for in these settings and are at greater risk of acquiring a healthcare associated infection (HAI). The Centers for Disease Control (CDC) has reported that most *Clostridium difficile* (*C. difficile*) infections are community acquired versus those that are acquired in a tertiary care settings (Voelker, 2012).

Healthcare associated infections (HAIs) continue to be of concern since their impact can be detrimental to patients (Marcel *et al.*, 2008). Three groups of microorganisms are primarily involved in HAIs. These

TABLE 8.1. Three Major Groups of Microorganisms and Percentage of HAI Cases.

Type of Microorganism	Examples of Microorganism	Percent of HAI Cases	How Disseminated
Commensal Bacteria	*Staphylococcus aureus* *Escherichia coli* *Enterococcus* spp	70–80%	Normal patient flora (skin, nasopharynx, feces) usually problematic during invasive procedures and spread on hands when introduced into sterile body sites
Saprophytic Bacteria	*Legionella* *Aspergillum* *P. aeruginosa* *Enterobacter* spp *Serratia* *Acinetobacter baumanni*	20–25%	Present in the environment (water, air, soil) and can colonize patients, particularly those receiving antibiotic therapy and case infections during invasive procedures. Other saprophytic agents can be spread through air or water
Highly Pathogenic Organisms	*Mycobacterium tuberculosis* Influenza virus Rotavirus Hepatitis B virus Hepatitis C virus	5%	Usually involved in epidemics in certain settings and can cause severe infections in very young and very old populations

include: *commensal bacteria, saprophytic bacteria,* and *highly pathogenic organisms* (Table 8.1).

8.3. CREATING THE CULTURE OF INFECTION CONTROL IN PRIMARY CARE SETTINGS

Regardless of the healthcare setting, HCPs must adhere to the basic principles associated with infection control. The foundational concepts for infection control and prevention must be patient-centered, based on best practice and meet the national or international guidelines for infection control. Creating a culture of infection control and prevention in primary care settings requires HCPs to understand the six foundational concepts of infection control:

1. All healthcare practices must be patient-centered, focusing on quality and safety.
2. Assessment of practice issues must adhere to the national and international principles of infection control.
3. Identification of and addressing systems of individual HCP issues related to poor or substandard infection control.
4. Continuously examining evidence-based practice standards for infection prevention and control and updating procedures/policies according to best practice.
5. Creating a culture of quality and safety in the healthcare setting by monitoring and performing surveillance related to the behavior of HCPs.
6. Rewarding HCPs who demonstrate excellence in modeling performance and outcomes of infection control practice.

These six foundational concepts provide a blueprint for an effective, timely, and relevant infection control and prevention program for primary care settings. Infection control programs have to be purposeful, consisting of comprehensive models at the micro-, macro-, and meso-system levels. They should additionally provide HCPs with benchmarks associated with accountability, monitoring, or rewards.

8.4. STRATEGIES FOR BEST PRACTICES FOR INFECTION CONTROL IN PRIMARY CARE SETTINGS

One of the greatest challenges to reduce the risk of HAIs in primary care settings is that these settings have traditionally lacked infection control surveillance (Centers for Disease Control and Prevention, 2011). In order to effect positive change and create a patient-centered culture of infection control in primary care settings, the practice model should focus on preventive strategies that interrupt the transmission of infections.

An infectious disease has the ability to be transmitted from person to person or spread through entire populations. The ability to spread is referred to as "*communicability*" (Merrill, 2013). The majority of infectious diseases are transmitted in primary care settings from one infected person to another through a process known as horizontal transmission. An example would be community-acquired methicillin-resistant Staphylococcus aureus (CA-MRSA), because it is related to skin-to-skin contact and its spread can occur quickly from person to person (Barnes and Sampson, 2011).

She also witnessed a healthcare provider perform an incision and drainage of an abscess on a patient that she suspected to have community-acquired methicillin-resistant Staphylococcus aureus (CA-MRSA).

The majorities of CA-MRSA infections occur as abscess(es), furuncles, or carbuncles in one site or multiple sites (Barnes and Sampson, 2011) and often are treated in primary care settings. Prior to treatment, it is important to obtain a culture from the drainage of the wound before a procedure or treatment. Care and handling of the equipment and the environment—including protection of the HCP with personal protective equipment (PPE)—is essential to meeting infection control standards.

The infection control model includes an understanding of the basic principles of epidemiology and an understanding of the chain of infection. It is important to interrupt the spread of potentially harmful microorganisms from patient to patient or from patient to HCP by interfering with the chain of infection.

8.4.1. Epidemiologic Model

The epidemiologic model represents the chain of infection and provides an interactive model representing the agent, host and environment. An epidemic or infectious process can be halted when one of the three major elements of the epidemiologic triad is interrupted. The agent relates to the causative, risk or environmental factors that may cause the infection. The host consists of the person or population that is affected by the infectious process. Last, the environment includes the place, characteristics, biological, physical, or psychosocial components that impact on the infectious process.

In the case of a primary care setting, the transmission of CA-MRSA can be prevented from spreading to a HCP or to a patient by initiating safe practices prior to the treatment of an incision and drainage (I & D) of a suspected CA-MRSA wound. The HCP should wear personal protective equipment (PPE) including a face shield, a fluid-resistant gown to cover the sleeves, and sterile gloves. Immediately after performing the I & D, the HCP should dispose of soiled or contaminated PPEs and immediately wash his/her hands with bactericidal cleansers. Additionally, the patient examination room should be properly cleansed prior to use for future patients. The epidemiological triad disrupts the chain of communicability and potential spread of the CA-MRSA through the prevention of horizontal disease transmission of highly contagious microorganisms (Centers for Disease Control and Prevention, 2006). The epidemiologic triad assists HCPs to determine best practice and strategies to break the chain of infection at any point between the agent, host or environment. In order for the infectious processes to exacerbate there must be a source of infection, a susceptible host, and a pathway for the microorganism to spread.

8.4.2. Source

The sources of infection are numerous and can be divided into two main groups: exogenous and endogenous sources. A source of infection is endogenous when the infectious agent comes from the patient's own body, usually from his own normal flora. Endogenous sources of infections become important when the person's own immunity against his normal flora becomes compromised such as in cases of contamination during surgery, malnutrition, impairment of blood supply and debilitating diseases such as AIDS, diabetes or any other accompanying infection. In the case of patients seeking care and treatment in primary care settings there may be many sources for infectious microorganisms (Table 8.2).

TABLE 8.2. *Major Sources and Reservoirs of Infectious Microorganisms and Mode of Transmission in Primary Care Settings.*

Major Sources of Infectious Microorganisms	Reservoirs	Examples of Mode of Transmission
Bacterial	Human and/or Inanimate Objects	Airborne, Personal Contact, Contaminated Countertops, Examination tables, Improperly cleansed or unsterilized equipment
Parasitic	Human	Person to person contact, improper hand washing, poor hygiene and hand to mouth contact
Viral	Human and/or Inanimate Objects	Airborne, Personal Contact, Contaminated Countertops, Examination tables, Improperly cleansed or unsterilized equipment
Fungal	Human and/or Inanimate Objects	Airborne, Personal Contact, Contaminated Countertops, Examination tables, Improperly cleansed or unsterilized equipment

8.4.3. Spread of Infection in Primary Care Settings

There are numerous pathways for microorganisms to spread in primary care settings. The major strategies to prevent the spread of microorganisms in these settings may be different than those used in acute-care settings where there is more infrastructure and monitoring of HCPs. For example, it is essential to make certain that no vials of medication or solutions are left in individual patient rooms. The use of multi dose vials or subscribing to unsafe injection practices may result in patient harm and transmission of infectious microorganisms to the host. HCPs need to monitor equipment and supplies more closely to prevent contamination of equipment between patients.

Lapses in infection control processes are reportedly the most common ways infectious microorganisms are transmitted to otherwise healthy patients. Patient-to-patient transmission of Hepatitis B and C viruses in primary care settings have been reported as a result of the contamination of multi-dose vials of injectable medications, flush solutions, reuse of finger stick devices intended for single patient use and the misuse of doses among multiple patients (Thompson *et al.*, 2009). HCPs in primary care settings need to be trained about the basic principles of infection control and adhere to the general standards of infection control to provide a safe environment for patient care.

Amy has always been accustomed to working in large tertiary care centers where someone else has had to worry about disinfection or the sterilization of instruments and monitoring infection control practices.

8.4.4. Proper Care and Cleaning of Medical Equipment

Wearing personal protective equipment (PPE) and routine cleaning of environmental surfaces between patients assist in the prevention of disease transmission. Meticulous attention to the types of cleaning procedures and products based on the manufacturers' recommendations has been suggested. For example, HCPs must adhere to the amount, dilution, contact time, safe use, ventilation, safety considerations, and proper disposal of product and types of cleaning products when disinfecting the patient's environment (Centers for Disease Control and Prevention, 2011). Use of these products provide a break in the chain of infection and provides a culture of safety for primary care patients (Table 8.3).

Medical equipment and supplies may be disposable or non-disposable, and it is critical to determine if medical equipment and supplies are intended for single or multiple patient use. It is imperative for HCPs in primary care settings to be knowledgeable and accountable for the proper use and care of either reusable or single use medical devices. The manufacturer must provide either reusable or single-use labels on medical equipment when it is purchased (Centers for Disease Control and Prevention, 2011).

8.4.5. Single Use Medical Equipment

Single use medical equipment usually refers to those medical devices that are for single patient use at one time, and are intended to be discarded after use. In primary care settings, the majority of the medical equipment such as finger sticks, needles, bandages, otoscope covers or plastic shields are examples of single use medical equipment. Finger lancets to prick the finger for blood samples to test for blood glucose for diabetic patients should never be reused. Use of the same lancet for different patients can result in a portal of entry for potential transmission of blood borne pathogens such as Hepatitis B or C. Sometimes HCPs may reuse single use devices and need to know the federal standards that are in place and what to do if breaches should occur (Table 8.4).

8.4.6. Reusable Medical Equipment

When reusable medical equipment is purchased, there are guidelines and instructions for cleaning for each specific piece of reusable medical equipment (Table 8.4, U.S. Food and Drug Administration, 2011). It is imperative that care involving cleaning and maintenance of reusable medical equipment follow manufacturers' guidelines and instructions to prevent and avoid patients being subjected to transmission of actual

TABLE 8.3. Recommended Process for Cleaning and Disinfection of Environmental Surfaces.

1. Evidence-based policies related to cleaning and disinfection for the environment.
2. Be certain that all employees are familiar with the policies for cleaning and disinfecting all equipment and patient rooms.
3. Monitor adherence by all employees within the primary care setting.
4. Select environmentally safe (Environmental Protection Agents) registered disinfectants or detergents with labels clearly indicating safe and effective use for healthcare settings.
5. Follow manufacturer's recommendations for safe and effective use in healthcare settings.

TABLE 8.4. FDA Regulatory Requirements for Reprocessing and Reuse of Single Use Medical Devices (U.S. Food and Drug Administration, 2009).

Reprocessing and reusing single-use devices (SUDs) can save costs and reduce medical waste.
Before medical devices can be reprocessed and reused, a third-party or hospital reprocessor must comply with the same requirements that apply to original equipment manufacturers, including: • Submitting documents for premarket notification or approval • Registering reprocessing firms and listing all products • Submitting adverse event reports • Tracking devices whose failure could have serious outcomes • Correcting or removing from the market unsafe devices • Meeting manufacturing and labeling requirements

or potentially infectious microorganisms (Centers for Disease Control and Prevention, 2008). *The CDC Guideline for Disinfection and Sterilization in Healthcare Facilities,* 2008 describes the history and process used to classify reusable instruments according to the Spaulding Classification System. The classification system was developed over 30 years ago specifically to clean, disinfect, and sterilize reusable medical instruments to decrease contamination and result in a safe, reusable medical object (CDC, 2008). The Spaulding Classification System classifies reusable medical devices as critical, semi critical, or noncritical based on contamination risk to the patient (Table 8.5). Additionally, the classification system provides examples of equipment, level of disinfection, and steps in the decontamination process.

Reusable medical equipment must be grounded in evidence-based procedures and policies that are readily available and known by all HCPs as part of the culture of safety and quality of the organization. HCPs must be educated and held accountable to uphold infection control and prevention practices in every patient encounter at all times.

8.4.7. Hand Hygiene

Use of good hand hygiene principles remains to be the single best way to interrupt the epidemiologic triad. Hand hygiene with plain or antimicrobial soap or hand gels is essential in containing or preventing spread of infectious disease in primary care settings. The use of proper techniques associated with safe hand hygiene promotes a model of quality and safety in these settings. Enforcement of infection control principles by all members of the healthcare team will assist in the

TABLE 8.5. Spaulding Classification of Medical Devices, Classification, Equipment, Disinfection and Decontamination Process.

Classification of Medical Device	Description of Classification	Example of Equipment	Level of Disinfection	Steps in the Decontamination Process
Low Risk (non critical item)	Items that come into contact with normal and intact skin	Stethoscopes, floor, walls, ceilings, furniture, sinks, etc.	Cleaning with detergent and drying is usually adequate	Clean, dry and store for future use
Intermediate Risk (semi-critical items)	Human and/or Inanimate Objects	Respiratory equipment, flexible endoscopes, laryngoscopes, specula, endotracheal tubes, thermometers, and other instruments	Cleaning followed by high level disinfectant (HLD) according to manufacture's guidelines	Clean, high level disinfectant or sterilization according to manufacturer's guidelines, dry and store
High Risk (critical items)	Items penetrating sterile body tissues including body cavities and vascular systems	Surgical instruments, intra-uterine devices, vascular catheters, impacts, etc.	Cleaning followed by manufacturer's sterilization guidelines	Clean, sterilize according to manufacturer's guidelines, dry and store

reduction of the transmission of infection from patient to patient or patient to HCP in the primary care setting.

8.5. SUMMARY POINTS

- Creating a culture of safety and quality for infection control in primary care settings
- Understanding the spread of infection in primary care settings
- Differentiation between disposable and reuse of medical equipment
- Standards associated with disinfection and sterilization
- Team efforts for preventing the spread of infection in primary care settings

8.6. REFERENCES

Barnes, B.E. and Sampson, D.A. (2011). A literature review on community-acquired methicillin-resistant Staphylococcus aureus in the United States: Clinical information for primary care nurse practitioners. *Journal of the American Academy of Nurse Practitioners, 23*: 23–32.

Centers for Disease Control and Prevention. (2006). Management of multi-resistant organisms in the healthcare settings. Retrieved from http://www.cdc.gov/hicpac/pdf/guidelines/MDROGuideline2006.pdf

Centers for Disease Control and Prevention. (2008). Guideline for Disinfection and Sterilization in healthcare facilities, 2008. Retrieved from http://www.cdc.gov/hicpac/Disinfection_Sterilization/20_00reference.html

Centers for Disease Control and Prevention. (2011). Guide to Infection Prevention for Outpatient Settings: Minimum Expectations for Safe Care, pp. 1–17. Retrieved from http://www.cdc.gov/HAI/pdfs/guidelines/standatds-of-primary care settings-care-7-2011.pdf

Centers for Disease Control and Prevention (2012). Diseases and Organisms in Healthcare Settings. Retrieved from http://www.cdc.gov/HAI/organisms/organisms.html

Marcel, J.P., Alpha, M., Baquero, F., et. al. (2008). Healthcare-associated infections: think globally, act locally. *Journal Compilation European Society of Clinical Microbiology and Infectious Diseases, 14*: 895–907.

Merrill, R. (2013). *Fundamentals of Epidemiology and Biostatistics: Combining the Basics.* Sudbury, MA: Jones & Bartlett.

Thompson, N.D., Perz, J.F., Moorman, A.C. and Holmberg, S.D. (2009). Nonhospital healthcare-associated Hepatitis B and C virus transmission: United States, 1998–2008. *American College of Physicians, 150*: 33–39.

U.S. Food and Drug Administration. (2009). Reprocessing Single Use Devices (SUDs). Retrieved from http://www.fda.gov/MedicalDevices/DeviceRegulationandGuidance/ReprocessingofSingle-UseDevices/default.htm

U.S. Food and Drug Administration. (2011). Processing Reusable Medical Devices.

Retrieved from http://www.fda.gov/MedicalDevices/DeviceRegulationandGuidance/ReprocessingofReusableMedicalDevices/default.htm

Voelker, R. (2012). Study: Vast majority of C. difficile infections occur in medical settings. *JAMA, 307*: 1356.

CHAPTER 9

Infection Control Principles for Long-term Care Environments

JUDITH SELTZER, RN, MS, CNOR and
DENISE M. KORNIEWICZ PhD., RN, FAAN

A realistic case study will be presented that includes a communicable disease typically found in patients who are in rehabilitation or long term care facilities. The major community acquired diseases or those most frequently encountered will be discussed. Approaches to the tracking, prevention of infection, precautions, and healthcare staff requirements will be presented. Other topics include wound care dressings, tube feedings, and use of catheters for urinary retention.

9.1. CASE PRESENTATION

It was the weekend and Kathy Jones was not looking forward to work on Monday. Over the past two weeks, three of the patients who reside in the long term care facility where Kathy worked became ill and were admitted to the hospital. Two patients returned to the facility diagnosed with staph infections. Just that morning while Kathy was getting ready for a family outing, she received a call from the center letting her know that another one of her residents was not doing well and the physician had been notified. For her part, Kathy spent most of the weekend reviewing resident charts, looking over staff documentation, staff continuing education programs and cleaning cycles of the facility. Some of the data she reviewed was somewhat shocking.

Kathy knew that her responsibility as the Director of Nursing was centered on the safe care for all residents. She also knew that in order to provide safe care for her residents she must also ensure that her staff is well educated on the guidelines of infection control and that education is an ongoing necessity based on maintaining an environment that will be free from external cross contamination as it relates to residents, staff and equipment.

141

When Kathy arrived at the facility on Monday morning, she saw an ambulance parked at the front door. When she entered, there was a lot of activity, as the charge nurse readied the paperwork that was to be sent to the hospital with the resident. This was patient number 4 and now even staff members are showing signs of worry. Kathy asked herself these questions: Is this the beginning of a facility-wide outbreak? What can be done to better protect the other residents and her staff from becoming infected?

Kathy determined that a complete review of infection prevention policies should be started immediately. Based on her weekend literature review, she already knew of some strategic measures that should be in the policies. Since HAIs must be monitored, audited, and reported in acute care settings, she should be initiating the same set of principles for the LTCF if they are not already included in policies. To assist in this initiative, Kathy will be seeking staff support and will form a facility-wide infection prevention team.

Kathy and her team will initiate closer links and identify a liaison between local hospitals associated with the facility. This liaison would serve to facilitate patient transfer between the various hospitals and the facility, and would increase awareness of infection prevention measures seen in both health care settings.

Kathy determined that education activities for her staff have been minimal. She now understands the importance of continuing education in infection prevention and will be addressing the facility Board of Directors to create a paid employee position to take the lead on infection prevention education. In addition to staff education, Kathy will implement more proficient infection prevention education for medical and non-medical personnel at her facility.

Kathy plans to review and, if warranted, revise the facility policy on antibiotic stewardship following best practice guidelines. Kathy, along with her leadership team, will continue to monitor appropriate nail care among her staff as well as that of the residents. Following the American Red Cross protocol for Geriatric Nursing Assistant (GNA) training requires successful completion of all designated skills prior to obtaining employment in this arena. (American Red Cross, 2010).

During her weekend reading, Kathy became well aware that more scientific work is needed around the issues of infection prevention in the LTCF. Previously, Kathy has never been approachable when asked to participate in research specifically geared towards the LTCF. After today, that will no longer be the case and Kathy will advocate to promote evidence based research in her facility on an ongoing basis.

Kathy understands that LTCFs are governed under guidelines set by the Joint Commission as well as the Centers for Medicare/ Medicaid, among others. To ensure a solid resolve and avoid additional outbreaks of *Staphylococcus aureus*, Kathy decides to meticulously review guidelines that may be appropriate for her facility.

9.2. ESSENTIAL CONTENT FOR INFECTION CONTROL SKILLS

After her arrival to the Center, Kathy decided to conduct an extensive literature review to better understand infection prevention-related trends that are currently seen in LTCFs across the country. She knows this would give her a better understanding moving forward with better infection prevention in her own facility.

In the United States, people are living longer due to advanced medical technologies. As more people age, the need for long term care facilities continue to increase as the mean age of the elderly has been reported to be 85 years old for women and 70 for men. Historically, long term care facilities (LTCFs), or nursing homes, typically housed elderly people with a chronic illness or simply individuals who had no one to care for them for the remainder of their lives. Today, this practice has changed, since LTCFs not only care for the elderly but care for younger patients needing short term rehabilitation or patients who are physically challenged.

Today, approximately 1.5 million persons currently reside in LTCFs across the country. Another 3 million people will enter a LTCF on a short term basis (http://www.aoa.gov/prof/Statistics/statistics.asp). This trend continues to increase, since patients require a higher level of nursing care and are being discharged earlier from acute care settings. Additionally, many short-term care patients are being discharged to LTCFs that include rehabilitation facilities following a surgical event. For example, recent orthopedic surgical patients who have undergone implant insertion may be discharged to a rehabilitation department and may be at risk for a surgical site infection due to transmission or cross contamination of pathogens. Because surgical site infections (SSIs) are one of the major complications related to orthopedic rehabilitation, the transfer of patients from an acute care facility to a LTCF must be closely monitored. Generally speaking, tracking of a hospital acquired infection (HAI) has not been monitored by LTCF personnel.

Historically, long term care facilities were centered on providing care for the aged and maintained use of basic or low technology. However, with the increasing acuity of medical and post-surgical patients in LTCFs, the clinical staff has had to adapt to multiple challenges to provide safe and effective patient care. This chapter will review current infection prevention guidelines associated with the ever-changing LTCF as well as discuss the need for good infection prevention guidelines for both short and long term residents.

9.2.1. Surveillance

In the United States, LTCFs report that 1.6 to 3.8 million infections occur each year. The overall infection rate in LTCFs for endemic infections ranges from 1.8 to 13.5 infections per 1000 resident-care days (Smith *et al.*, 2008). Because of these statistics, healthcare providers, as well as patient family members, view infections as expected or common among residents of LTCFs (Nicolle, 2000). The three most common outbreaks among residents in LTCFs include respiratory, urinary tract, and skin or soft tissue infections. Diligent surveillance for these common outbreaks includes monitoring for the clinical symptoms associated with the type of infection (Table 9.1).

Elderly patients in LTCFs tend to be more susceptible to outbreaks of infection of colonizing organisms due to their close proximity to other patients as well as the overriding amount of visitors to the facility on a daily basis. Therefore, use of an accepted standard of care related to infection control among staff, patients and visitors can decrease the incidence and prevalence of HAIs in the LTCF. An effective infection prevention program targeted for the LTCF population enhances patient safety and assures that quality patient care is provided.

9.2.2. Implementation of Standard Precautions

When Kathy sets about to review the facility protocols concerning infection control, she becomes acutely aware that standard precautions and methodologies need to become commonplace regardless of any outbreak of an infection within the facility.

TABLE 9.1. Surveillance for Types of Infection and Body Site among Residents in LTCF.

Type of Infection	Criteria	Clinical Symptoms
Upper Respiratory	Common Cold	Runny nose, sneezing, sore throat, hoarseness, difficulty swallowing, dry couth, fever, tender glands
	Ear	Drainage, diagnosis of ear infection
	Mouth	Mouth infection diagnosed by dentist
	Sinusitis	Diagnosed and receiving antibiotics
	Influenza-like illness	Chills, headache, muscle aching, malaise, loss of appetite, sore throat, fever
Lower Respiratory	Pneumonia	Positive chest x-ray for infiltrate
		Cough, sputum production, chest pain, wheezing, rhonchi, shortness of breath
Urinary Tract	Without Catheter	Fever, chills, burning on urination, frequency, urgency, flank pain, tenderness, incontinence
	With Catheter	Fever, chills, suprapubic pain, tenderness, change in mental or functional status
Skin & Soft tissue	Presence of wound	Pus, fever, heat, redness, tenderness, swelling

Standard precautions are measures that must be used in caring for all persons in every healthcare setting. They are designed to prevent the transmissions of microorganisms and blood borne viruses between patients/residents, staff and visitors, irrespective of whether it is known that the person/patient does or does not have a communicable infection (Smith *et al.*, 2008; AORN, 2011; Flanagan *et al.*, 2011). These standard practices include adherence to hand hygiene practices by staff and visitors, use of protective equipment, environmental controls, and use of infection control guidelines.

Hand hygiene includes hand washing and the use of antiseptic hand gels. Traditional hand washing should be done when the hands are visibly soiled or after patient care. The use of antiseptic hand gels is appropriate before and after patient contact as long as the heathcare provider's (HCP) hands are not visibly soiled. Hand hygiene must be carried out correctly before and after direct contact with patients/clients, contact with their immediate environment and contaminated items (e.g., commodes or dirty laundry). Additionally, good hand hygiene principles should be used after removing personal protective clothing, including gloves.

9.2.2.1. Hand Hygiene Issues for Staff

Hand Hygiene issues for staff include guidelines associated with the use of artificial fingernails. Several studies have demonstrated that healthcare personnel using artificial nails may harbor infectious pathogens under their artificial nails. For example, the use of artificial nails can result in carrying Gram-negative organisms and yeast (HICPAC/SHEA/APIC/IDSA Hand Hygiene Task Force, 2002). Therefore, it has been recommended that healthcare providers, patient care extenders, and family members who provide care to patients not wear artificial nails. Additionally, natural nails should be kept short (approximately 1/4 inch long) to prevent the transmission of gram negative pathogens from provider to patient (HICPAC/SHEA/APIC/IDSA Hand Hygiene Task Force, 2002).

9.2.2.2. Hand Hygiene Issues for Patients

Hand hygiene issues for patients/client continue to be of concern, since the patient or resident may also be a vector for an infectious pathogen. Patient fingernails should be manicured, which includes cleaning, cutting and filing on a regular basis. Patients will be at higher risk for skin and soft tissue infections (MRSA) if pathogens are allowed to be harbored under the nail beds, allowing the patient to serve as their own reservoir for infection.

Whether it is a healthcare provider, patient or visitor, proper implementation of hand hygiene remains the most effective and least expensive measure to prevent transmission of pathogenic organisms in a health care setting. Despite continued education efforts to improve hand hygiene in facilities, compliance with hand hygiene remains dismal, averaging only 30% to 50% among healthcare providers. (HICPAC/SHEA/APIC/IDSA Hand Hygiene Task Force, 2002). Healthcare facility administrators must continue to enforce hand hygiene guidelines and provide surveillance information to their employees. However, both the consumer and the patients must be educated and advocate for adherence to these policies.

9.2.2.3. Wearing Jewelry during Patient Care

Wearing jewelry during patient care continues to be of concern. Several studies have demonstrated an increased presence of colonization of pathogenic organisms under rings compared to other areas of the hand without rings (HICPAC/SHEA/APIC/IDSA Hand Hygiene Task Force, 2002). Rings with rough surfaces may remain dirty in crevices after washing hands. Rings may also tear gloves and may possibly injure patients during care. In general, a consensus recommendation to health-care setting administrators has been to strongly discourage healthcare providers and visitors from wearing rings or other jewelry while providing patient care (WHO, 2009).

9.2.2.4. Appropriate Use of Personal Protective Equipment, Which Includes Gloves, Aprons, Gowns, Face and Eye Protection

Gloves and sometimes aprons must be used when in contact with blood or body fluids, secretions, excretions and contaminated items (e.g., the commode, soiled linen, or dressings). Gloves must be discarded immediately following use, changed between patients, and hand hygiene is essential after the removal of gloves. If there is a risk of blood or body fluid splashes, masks and eye protection should be used.

9.2.2.5. Appropriate Handling and Disposal of Waste and Disposal of Sharps

Waste must always be disposed of into the appropriate bag or container. Sharps must be disposed of directly into a sharps box and infected or blood stained waste into a clinical waste bin or bag. Incontinence waste such as diapers and empty urine bags not contaminated with blood should be disposed of as household waste. Disposable gloves must be worn when handling waste. Gloves must be disposed of and hand hygiene performed following the handling of waste.

9.2.2.6. Appropriate Handling and Management of Clean and Used Linen

Clean linen should be stored in a clean dry area. Dirty linen should be handled with care and disposed of in the appropriate linen bags. Soiled linens should be stored in a clean dry area to await collection for transfer to the laundry.

9.2.2.7. Appropriate Decontamination of the Environment and Healthcare Equipment

The healthcare environment must be visibly clean, free from dust and spills, and be acceptable to the clients/patients, visitors, and staff. Reusable equipment must not be used for the care of another patient/ client until it has been decontaminated and reprocessed appropriately. Single use items must not be reused and must be discarded appropriately according to manufacturers' instructions.

9.2.2.8. Suitable Placement of Patients

The isolation of a nursing home resident to prevent the spread of HAIs is common and should be routine, as the risk of spreading a serious infection may be just as serious as in an acute care hospital. However, when a single room is not available, an infected patient (Administration on Aging, 2010) may sometimes be placed with patients or clients infected by the same microorganism, provided they are not infected with other potentially transmissible microorganisms. Such sharing of rooms, also referred to as cohorting, is useful, especially during outbreaks or when there is a shortage of single rooms. However, the overall needs of the patient or resident must take precedence when attempting to limit the spread of infection through isolation or cohorting.

9.2.2.9. Respiratory Hygiene and Cough Etiquette

Measures should be taken to contain respiratory secretions. Advise patients to cover their mouth and nose with a disposable tissue when coughing or sneezing and dispose of the tissue promptly into the waste bin. Hand hygiene after contact with respiratory secretions is essential to prevent infection spreading. Staff should ensure that supplies of tissues, waste bins and hand hygiene facilities are available.

9.2.2.10. Transport of Laboratory Specimens

The transport of laboratory specimens should follow the occupational safety and health agency's (OSHA) guidelines to minimize contamination or the spread of an infectious substance. In order to minimize the cross-transfer of microorganisms from patient to patient or patient to healthcare provider, it is best to minimize the direct handling of specimens by using sealable plastic bags or closed system culture containers. Use of a standardized method to collect the laboratory specimen as well as the proper method of transportation assists in the reduction of possible infectious outbreaks within a LTCF (Table 9.2.).

TABLE 9.2. Procedure for Collecting and Transporting Laboratory Specimens.

Type of Culture	Anatomic Site	Procedure
Nasal	Anterior nares	Use nasal swab from culturette container and crush ampoule to ensure swab remains wet
Throat	Throat	Swab back of throat in tonsillar area using culturette container
Skin	Anatomical area of infected surface	Scrap skin into sterile, screw cap container
Sputum	Immediately following cough	Have resident cough and spit into sterile screw cap container
Ear	Ear drainage from infected ear	Use swab from culturette
Eye	Eye drainage from infected eye	Use swab from culturette
Wounds or abscesses	Surface wounds	Use sterile saline moistened gauze to remove accumulated purulent drainage and insert into sterile specimen container
	Abscesses	Use needle and syringe to aspirate fluid; transfer contents to sterile container
Urine	Clean, voided or catheter	Collect in sterile container, note date and time of collection
Feces	Collect stool	Use fecal transport media; if *C. difficile*, follow lab manual to assure accurate collection media; note date and time of collection
Blood cultures	Venipuncture	Use steps outlined for obtaining blood cultures. Specimens should be drawn 1/2 hour apart for a total of 3 within a 24 hr. period
Intravascular (IV) catheters	Note anatomical site	Aseptically remove catheter; with sterile scissors, clip 5 cm of the distal tip of catheter and put in sterile container

9.2.2.11. Immunizations

Current recommendations by the CDC has recommended that both patients and HCPs obtain specific seasonal immunizations for communicable diseases. The immunizations that have been regulated and or mandated include influenza vaccines, tetanus, or tuberculosis screening.

9.2.2.12. Transfer of Residents

Over the past two weeks, three of the patients who reside in the long term care facility where Kathy worked became ill and were admitted to the hospital. Two patients returned to the facility diagnosed with staph infections.

Kathy and her team will initiate closer links and identify a liaison between local hospitals associated with the facility. This liaison would serve to facilitate patient transfer between the various hospitals and the facility, increasing awareness of infection prevention measures seen in both health care settings.

Transfer protocols between acute care and LTCF need to be in place to track and identify any potential communicable disease exposure. Open communication between facilities permitting the exchange of information about the resident should include information such as pertinent clinical data, medical history, presenting signs or symptoms of infections, appropriate culture reports and antibiotic therapy. Specific information related to the history of any multiple resistant organisms or risk factors associated with the colonization of pathogenic organisms need to be disclosed. Use of a transfer form with specific categories related to potential communicable diseases has been recommended by CDC.

9.2.2.13. Common Infectious Disease Outbreaks

Outbreaks of infection are common in LTCF and have been reported to include a variety of organisms. Because of the variables that impact on institutional patients such as functional impairment, co-morbidities and chronic disease, the risk of infection in residents may be greater than in other health care settings. Efforts to prevent the transmission of infection between residents is the primary catalyst to infection control policies. However, in spite of such efforts, some common endemic outbreaks include a higher incidence of colonization with antimicrobial-resistant organisms, including methicillin-resistant *Staphylococcus aureus* (MRSA). Often patients acquire MRSA in the acute care facility and remain colonized for extended periods, even when transferred to a LTCF. There is no evidence to support the non-admission of residents to a LTCF on the basis of being colonized or infected by resistant organisms. In fact, the use of antimicrobials in LTCF has been ineffective and has not decreased the incidence of MRSA (Table 9.3).

Often co-morbidities such as impairment of functional status has been highly associated with asymptomatic bacteriuria resulting from bowel and bladder incontinence. The use of indwelling or condom catheters may be useful in some patients; however, avoidance of the use

TABLE 9.3. Top CDC Recommendations; MRSA (CDC, 2011).

To Prevent MRSA Infections:
• Comply with CDC hand hygiene recommendations
• Implement Contact Precautions for MRSA colonized and infected patients
• Recognize previously MRSA colonized and infected patients
• Rapidly report MRSA lab results
• Provide MRSA education for healthcare providers
Also consider:
• Active surveillance testing—screening of patients to detect colonization even if no evidence of infection
• Other novel strategies
— Decolonization
— Chlorhexidine bathing

of these devices has been recommended (Table 9.4). Additionally, the use of catheterization for managing bladder training or voiding demonstrated higher rates of urinary tract infections (Duffy, 1995).

Clostridium difficile continues to be a major cause of infectious diarrhea, with reported rates ranging from 1–10 cases per 1000 discharges among elderly patients in LTCF (Simor *et al.*, 2002). The symptoms associated with the organism may cause severe, even life-threatening disease and has caused outbreaks in LTCF. Antibiotic-associated diarrhea is common among LTCF residents with over 33% of LTCF residents having been found to have acquired *C. difficile* within 2 weeks of antimicrobial therapy. Outbreaks of *C.difficile* have attributed the transmis-

TABLE 9.4. Top CDC Recommendations to Prevent Healthcare Associated Infections.

To Prevent Catheter-Associated Urinary Tract Infections (CAUTIs):
• Insert catheters only for appropriate indications
• Leave catheters in place only as long as needed
• Ensure that only properly trained persons insert and maintain catheters
• Insert catheters using aseptic technique and sterile equipment (acute care setting)
• Follow aseptic insertion, maintain a closed drainage system
• Maintain unobstructed urine flow
• Comply with CDC hand hygiene recommendations and Standard Precautions
Also consider:
• Alternatives to indwelling urinary catheterization
• Use of portable ultrasound devices for assessing urine volume to reduce unnecessary catheterizations
• Use of antimicrobial/antiseptic-impregnated catheters

sion of the organism to the hands of personnel, fomites or the nursing home environment (Brooks *et al.*, 1992; Fawley and Wilcox, 2001). HCPs may also contribute to the spread of *C.difficile* during an outbreak by assisting patients in using contaminated commodes or equipment, or by touching contaminated surfaces themselves, such as telephones.

9.3. GENERAL ENVIRONMENTAL ISSUES (WHEELCHAIRS, HAND RAILS, WALKERS, CLEANING ROOMS)

Kathy determined that education activities for her staff have been minimal. She now understands the importance of continuing education in infection prevention and will be addressing the facility Board of Directors to include a paid employee position to take the lead on education. In addition to staff education, Kathy will implement more proficient infection prevention education for medical training and of training for non-medical personnel at her facility.

Implementation of infection control programs include the identification of environmental issues that impact on the transmission of microorganisms that may cause an infectious outbreak. Specifically in LTCF, staff need to be aware of environmental conditions that may directly or indirectly contribute to a possible infectious outbreak. Since administrators of LTCFs following the vision of CMS, strive to promote a home-like environment, the challenges include prevention techniques that impact on the staff as well as the residents. For example, use of hand gels in between patient care, cleaning walkers, wheelchairs, assistive de-

TABLE 9.5. Appropriate Times to Wash Your Hands in a LTCF.

Appropriate Times to Wash Your Hands in the Long Term Care Facility:
• Coming on Duty and When Leaving the Facility
• Whenever Hands are Visibly Soiled
• Personal Use of Toilet
• After Contact with any Resident Secretions
• Performing any Invasive Procedures
• Leaving a Resident's Isolation Room
• After Handling Items such as Bedpans, Dressings, Catheters
• After Removing Gloves
• Before and After any Personal Meals
• Allowing the Resident Time and Means to Wash Their Hands Before and After Meals

vices and handrails may decrease the spread of infections (Appendix A). The management of infections must be refocused since residents are immuno-suppressed and few advancements have been made within their setting (Smith *et al.*, 2008).

No policy, protocol or guideline is more important than that of hand hygiene. The facility's handwashing policy should be clear and concise and staff should expect that the policy will be monitored (Table 9.5).

A 20-second handwash is recommended using friction with a chemical agent. If the facility cannot provide adequate sinks where appropriate handwashing can take place, then the facility must provide alcohol based handrubs (Smith *et al.*, 2008).

9.4. REGULATORY MEASURES

Kathy understands that LTCFs are governed under guidelines set by the Joint Commission of Accreditation and Association of periOperative Registered Nurses,and Centers for Medicare/Medicaid to name a few. To ensure a solid resolve and avoid additional outbreaks of Staphylococcal aureus, Kathy decides to review guidelines that may be appropriate for her facility.

In 2011, Joint Commission Long Term Care National Patient Safety Goals were announced. Table 9.6. provides the regulatory goals that have been recommended.

Based on these regulations, all LTCF have an obligation to adhere to the standards and provide safe and effective care for patients, staff and family members.

9.5. SUMMARY POINTS

- HAIs in LTCFs need to be monitored
- Consistent surveillance for endemic infections in LTCFs is a necessity
- Use of the CDC's hand hygiene guidelines is recommended for LTCFs
- Monitoring the patient's environment is an evidence based strategy for LTCFs
- Use of personal protective equipment which includes gloves, gowns, face and eye protection is recommended
- Safe handling and disposal of waste and sharps

- Safe handling and management of clean and used linen, which includes the patients' clothes
- Decontamination of the environment with documentation is recommended for safe patient environments (Appendix A)
- Suitable placement of patients to reduce the transmission of infection is recommended
- Respiratory hygiene and cough etiquette
- Occupational health—vaccines are recommended
- Skin de-colonization with the use of a 4% CHG solution for patient bathing

TABLE 9.6. Joint Commission Accreditation Long Term Care National Patient Safety Goals, 2011.

The purpose of the National Patient Safety Goals is to improve patient safety. The goals focus on problems in health care safety and how to solve them.	
Identify residents correctly NPSG.01.01.01	Use at least two ways to identify residents. For example, use the resident's name and date of birth. This is done to make sure that each resident gets the correct medicine and treatement.
Use medicines safely NPSG.03.05.01	Take extra care with patients who take medicines to thin their blood.
NPSB.03.06.01	Record and pass along correct information about a resident's medicines. Find out what medicines the resident is taking. Compare those medicines to new medicines given to the resident. Make sure the resident knows which medicines to take when they are at home. Tell the resident it is important to bring their up-to-date list of medicines every time they visit a doctor.
Prevent Infection NPSG.07.01.01	Use the hand cleaning guidelines from the Centers for Disease Control and Prevention or the World Health Organization. Set goals for improving hand cleaning. Use the goals to improve hand cleaning.
NPSG.07.04.01	Use proven guidelines to prevent infection of the blood from central lines.
Prevent residents from falling NPSG.09.02.01	Find out which residents are most likely to fall. For example, is the resident taking any medicines that might make them weak, dizzy or sleepy? Take action to prevent falls for htese residents.
Prevent bed sores NPSG.14.01.01	Find out which residents are most likely to have bed sores. Take action to prevent bed sores in these patients. From time to time, re-check residents for bed sores.

Appendix A: Daily High Touch Cleaning Checklist
Environmental Cleaning
Daily Cleaning of High Touch Areas

*Unit:*_____

Date: _____

Area	Yes	No	Comments/Reason Area Not Cleaned	Initials
Doorknobs				
Bedrails				
Light Switches				
Overbed Tables				
Phone				
Remote Control				
Bedside Cabinet				
Bathroom Sink Faucet				
Toilet Handle				
Call Light				

*Checklist that could be used by LTCF to monitor daily environmental cleaning.

9.6. REFERENCES

Administration on Aging. Statistics on the Aging Population. Available at http://www.aoa.gov/prof/Statistics/statistics.asp. Accessed August 2010.

American Red Cross. (2011). GNA Candidates LTCF Skills Training.

AORN. (2011) Perioperative standards and recommended practices. Preventable Transmission of Infections in the Perioperative Practice Setting, pp. 291–301.

Brooks, S.E., Veal, R.O., Kramer, M., *et al.* (1992) Reduction in the incidence of Clostridium difficile-associated diarrhea in an acute care hospital and a skilled nursing facility following replacement of electronic thermometers with single-use disposables. *Infect. Control Hosp. Epidemiol., 13*:98–103.

Centers for Disease Control and Prevention (CDC) (2011). Top CDC Recommendations to Prevention Healthcare Associated Infections.

Duffy, L.M., Cleary, J., Ahern, S., *et al.* (1995) Clean intermittent catheterization: Safe, cost-effective bladder management for male residents of VA nursing homes. *J. Am. Geriatr. Soc. 43*:865-70.

Fawley, W.N. and Wilcox, M.H. (2001) Molecular epidemiology of endemic Clostridium difficile infection. *Epidemiol. Infect., 126*:343–350.

Flanagan, E., et al. (2011) Infection prevention in alternative care settings. *Infect. Dis. Clin. N. AM. 25*: 271–283.

HICPAC/SHEA/APIC/IDSA Hand Hygiene Task Force. (2002) Guideline for hand hygiene in health-care settings: recommendations of the Healthcare Infection Control Practices Advisory Committee and the HICPAC/SHEA/APIC/

IDSA Hand Hygiene Task Force. MMWR Recomm Rep. 51(RR16):1–45. Available at: http://www.cdc.gov/ncidod/dhqp/g1_handhygiene.html

Joint Commission Accreditation Long Term Care. (2011). Long Term Care National Patient Safety Goals.

Nicolle, L. (2000) Infection Control in Long Term Care Facility. Special Section Healthcare Epidemiology. *Clinical Infectious Diseases 31*:752–756.

Simor A.E., Bradley, S.F., Strausbaugh, L.J., *et al.* (2002) Clostridium difficile in long-term-care facilities for the elderly. *Infect. Control Hosp. Epidemiol. 23*(11):696–703.

Smith, P., *et al.* (2008) SHEA/APIC Guideline: Infection prevention and control in the long term care facility. *Amer. J. Infec. Control 36*:504–535.

WHO. Guidelines on Hand Hygiene in Health Care. Patient Safety. Geneva: World Health Organization. Practical issues and potential barriers to optimal hand hygiene practices, p.132.

CHAPTER 10

Infection Control in the Home

JEANETTE ADAMS, PhD., RN, ACNS-BC, CRNI

*The purpose of this chapter is to discuss infection control principles en-
countered in the home environment. An example of a complicated case
study about a patient who is at risk for infection due to immune suppres-
sion and multiple risk factors will be presented. Topics will include the
need to teach care providers about the types of environmental issues that
impact on homecare patients.*

10.1. CASE PRESENTATION

Pamela Harrison is a home health nurse who works with
America Home Health, a national comprehensive home care
agency. American Home Health provides services within a ra-
dius of 250 miles from the regional office. Client referrals are
received on a continuous basis from a variety of acute health
care facilities in the region. Pamela is the admissions coordinator. She is responsible for providing initial assessments for new
clients and conducts a home care visit to transition the client
from care at an acute care facility to care at their home setting.

During lunch, Pamela receives notification from Southern
Medical Center, a regional acute care facility, that Juanita Gonzalez is being discharged home this afternoon. Pamela receives
information from the acute care nurse so that she can prepare
for the visit at Mrs. Gonzalez's home. The care coordinator informs Pamela that Mrs. Gonzalez is a 58 year-old female, who is
being discharged from the hospital following post-operative abdominal surgery related to colon cancer. She contracted a health
care-associated infection post operatively and was started on an
antibiotic regimen with a peripherally inserted central catheter

157

(PICC). She was also placed on parenteral nutrition with a central venous catheter to allow bowel rest and provide caloric intake. Mrs. Gonzalez has a secondary diagnosis of Type II diabetes and uses Insulin to control her blood glucose. She is required to check her blood glucose before meals. A foley urinary catheter was inserted post operatively because of urinary retention and is to remain for bladder training. Mrs. Gonzalez has incidents of stool incontinence. During her hospitalization, Juanita was found to have multidrug resistant organisms (MDRO), including methicillin-resistant Staphylococcus aureus (MRSA).

America Home Health is responsible for coordinating Mrs. Gonzalez's care in the home setting for her incisional wound, parenteral nutrition, antibiotic therapy, blood work, pain management, blood glucose control and urinary care. America Home Health will provide intermittent nursing care, medical supplies and pharmaceutical medications and solutions to the home. Pamela will provide an initial assessment for admission and schedule future visits for care and evaluation.

Pamela schedules a time to meet with Mr. and Mrs. Gonzalez at their home later in the day. Pamela travels to the client's home in her personal car, which is a sport utility vehicle (SUV). She carries medical disposable supplies in a plastic container in the back portion of the SUV. She also carries a nylon nurse's bag containing her stethoscope, sphygmomanometer, and other small physical assessment apparatus along with disposable medical supplies, hand hygiene solution, forms and pens. Pamela wears a scrub suit with a lab coat. On an annual basis, Pamela provides documented evidence of tuberculosis skin test, hepatitis B immunization, an update of infection control and prevention policies and procedures and certification of cardiopulmonary resuscitation.

Pamela determines that Mrs. Gonzalez lives approximately 60 miles from the home care office and it will take her an hour and a half to drive to the house. Pamela carries a cell telephone for communication to the home and the office and a global positioning system to assist in locating the Gonzalez's house with the home address and written directions. These tools offer Pamela safety as well as keep her connected to the office and client.

Upon arrival at Mrs. Gonzalez's home, Pamela realizes that the house is on an unpaved road and that the nearest other home is one mile away. The house is located in a rural area in the South surrounded by farms. This is the beginning of Pamela's home assessment. Mr. and Mrs. Gonzalez have been home two hours prior to Pamela's arrival. This gives them time to get settled into their home surroundings before Pamela's appointment.

As Pamela parks her car, there are several feral cats and dogs as well as chickens that greet her. Pamela gets out of the car and retrieves her nylon nurse's bag before entering Mrs. Gonzalez's home. Mr. Gonzalez meets Pamela at the front door and invites her into the house. Mrs. Gonzalez is in the bed in the bedroom she shares with her husband.

Pamela meets Mr. and Mrs. Gonzalez and ensures that Mrs. Gonzalez is comfortable before she begins her admission process and starts a medical health record. Pamela conducts assessments of the home environment, family and social network and caregiver support. Mrs. Gonzalez lives in a one-story, three bedroom and one bathroom house with her husband, Gorge, her son, Gorge, Jr., and his two children, ages 8 and 10. There are pets consisting of two cats and one dog that live in the house. The house does not have central climate control, but has one window air conditioning unit in the family room. The bedrooms and kitchen have electric fans for ventilation. A well supplies the water source and the house has plumbing and one toilet. Her daughter, Maria, lives out of state with her family. Gorge, Jr. works on the farm with his father. The children attend public school during the day. Ordinarily, Mrs. Gonzalez cares for the children. Mrs. Gonzalez's husband, Gorge, works as a farmer. He has a ninth-grade education and Spanish is his primary language. There are chickens in the yard and cows in the pasture next to the house. The farm has crops of corn and other vegetables. There are several feral cats and dogs around the house.

Since Mrs. Gonzalez receives intermittent home care nursing visits and not around the clock nursing care, she and her family are responsible for maintenance of her care. Pamela begins patient and family education of the plan of care at home. Pamela conducts an internal home assessment to determine environmental safety and conduciveness to home care.

10.2. ESSENTIAL CONTENT FOR INFECTION CONTROL SKILLS

Home health care presents many challenges as a setting for health care. In institutional health care facilities, health care workers have control over the environmental work areas with resources such as house-keeping, infection control personnel and supportive departments to ensure patient safety and infection prevention measures. Home health care is an autonomous practice setting where great variations of practice occur (Kenneley, 2007). Of the estimated 8 million home care patients, approximately 1.2 million infections occur in the home care setting (Mannagan et al., 2002). High risk patients for infection receiving home care include those receiving the following procedures: (1) intravascular access, especially central lines; (2) mechanical ventilation; (3) surgical drains; (4) parenteral nutrition; (5) urinary tract instrumentation, especially indwelling catheterization; and (6) extracorporeal membrane oxygenation. (Kenneley, 2007). Adherence to measures of infection prevention and control can reduce the infection risk in home care. The purpose of this chapter will be to discuss infection control principles encountered in the home environment.

Upon arrival at Mrs. Gonzalez's home, Pamela realizes that the house is on an unpaved road and that the nearest other home is one mile away. The house is located in a rural area in the South surrounded by farms. This is the beginning of Pamela's home assessment. As Pamela parks her car, there are several feral cats and dogs as well as chickens that greet her. Mrs. Gonzalez is in the bed in the bedroom she shares with her husband. Mrs. Gonzalez lives in a one-story, three bedroom and one bathroom house with her husband, Gorge, her son, Gorge, Jr., and his two children, ages 8 and 10. There are pets consisting of two cats and one dog that live in the house. The house does not have central climate control, but has one window air conditioning unit in the family room. The bedrooms and kitchen have electric fans for ventilation. A well supplies the water source and the house has plumbing and one toilet.

10.2.1. Home Environment

Whenever a patient is discharged for home care, a home assessment must be conducted. An assessment is necessary to evaluate the safety and appropriateness of the home as a setting for the care of the patient. The home assessment includes sources of electricity, water, plumbing, toilets and bathrooms, space, communication availability and cleanliness. Accessibility for the patient is another consideration. The patient needs someone to assist as a caregiver. This most often includes a family member who is also living in the household, but may also involve social and community support.

10.2.2. Hygiene

Hand hygiene is the single most important prevention activity that reduces the transmission of infectious agents. The patient and family must be taught the importance of hand washing, especially before and after providing care to the patient to decrease cross contamination. The home care nurse must also practice vigilant hand washing behavior in the care of the patient. The home care nurse should be sure to use hand hygiene upon entering the home and prior to leaving the home. The home care nurse should not use the bar soap or multiuse towels provided in the patient's home. The nurse should bring her/his own liquid soap and paper towels for hand hygiene. When water is not available, the nurse should use the alcohol based rubs as directed by the manufacturer (Felemban *et al.*, 2012).

10.2.3. Disinfection

Cleanliness of the home is part of the home assessment. It is evident whenever the home is insect and/or rodent infested (Clark, 2010). However, neatness does not always indicate cleanliness (Kenneley, 2012). The home environment promotes transmission of infections through household items such as vacuum bags, refrigerators, countertops, soil, and cutting boards. Contamination may occur from family contact, inanimate objects and pets (Cozad *et al.*, 2003). Poor housing conditions and inadequate use of disinfectants can also contribute to the potential risk of transmission of infections. Germicidal detergents are essential for disinfection when patients with infections receive care at home. The home environment is a reservoir for growth of pathogens. Disinfection removes most pathogenic microorganisms on inanimate objects. Chemical disinfectants such as alcohol, chlorine compounds, hydrogen peroxide, phenolics, quaternary ammonium compounds, and iodophors can be used in the home setting (McGoldrick, 2010). Antiseptics are used on living tissue (OSHA, 2001).

10.2.4. Clothing

The Occupational and Safety Health Administration (OSHA) clearly distinguishes between soiled clothing such as scrubs and contaminated clothing. Clothing that is worn may be soiled by perspiration, body oils or any other items that the nurse may come in contact with during the course of their work. Contamination, on the other hand, refers to clothing that must have come in contact with blood or other potentially infectious materials. If clothing is contaminated, it should be removed without contaminating other items and placed separately in a plastic bag for laundering (OSHA, 2001). Home care workers should always carry extra clothing in the event of contamination or wear paper gowns when the probability of contamination exists, such as in wound care or blood drawing. Personal protective equipment (PPE) is a standard of practice in home care as in any other health care setting (Leiss *et al.*, 2011). PPE is used with the possibility of blood and body fluid contact that may include, but is not limited to, dressing changes, patients with HIV, viral encephalitis and Hepatitis B, C, D, and E (Rhinehart and McGoldrick, 2006).

10.2.5. Laundry

Laundry procedures should include washing in warm water with detergent and sanitizer or chlorine bleach and placing in a dryer. There is no scientific evidence that home laundry contributes to the transmission of infectious agents (Belkin, 2001). Jurkovich (2004) found no pathogenic growth on home-laundered scrubs ($n = 20$). In contrast, Wiener-Well *et al.* (2011) isolated pathogens from 63% of health care worker uniforms in an acute care setting with 14% isolated antibiotic resistant bacteria. The role of transmission of pathogens to clients has not been determined. Bedclothes that risk contamination with blood and body fluids should also be laundered in warm water with detergent and sanitizer and placed in a dryer.

10.2.6. Space

Not all households have adequate space conducive to home health care. Most home care patients require medical equipment, disposable medical supplies and pharmaceutical agents. Home care providers provide deliveries of these items in various time frames ranging from a week to a month. This determines how much medical storage is needed. A clean area in the home away from the possibility of liquid penetration must be dedicated for the storage area of medical supplies to maintain the integrity of the products. Some supplies, such as pharmaceutical agents, may require refrigeration. A thermometer needs to be placed in the refrigerator and monitored to ensure the proper temperature for the duration of storage. Supplies need to be stored in a cool, dry area away from direct sunlight.

10.2.7. Sharps Container

A sharps container must be provided and used only for sharps disposal. Sharps should be directly placed in the sharps container immediately after use. It is necessary to store the sharps container in an area away from pets and children. Sharps should not be disposed in household containers or in household waste. Bloodborne transmission of infection is high risk with the use of contaminated sharps.

10.2.8. Climate Control

Uncontrolled climate control environments increase the potential risk of infections by providing a medium of growth for microorganisms in perspiration, especially during high temperatures. Open windows and use of fans for ventilation allow the circulation of dust from the outside environment into the home interior. Vectors such as flies, ticks and mosquitoes are also allowed to enter the inner domain of the home, leading to the potential transmission of infections. The presence of pets and animals increase the affinity of vectors entering the household.

10.3. HEALTH CARE PROVIDERS

Home health care providers involve many personnel and services to the patient. Storage and delivery of disposable medical supplies, equipment and pharmaceutical agents are all part of the continuum of care for the patient receiving home care.

10.3.1. Transportation

Inherent in home health care is transportation of goods to the patient's residence. Temperature impacts the quality of the supplies during transport. Medical supplies and pharmaceutical agents generally have a range of temperature to uphold. Whenever temperatures vary outside these safety ranges, product deterioration begins. Climate controlled delivery vehicles are imperative to ensure the efficacy and safety of supplies and pharmaceuticals. The health care worker also uses a vehicle to transport supplies and pharmaceutical agents. Unlike the delivery vehicle that is used primarily for scheduled deliveries, the health care worker's car is parked for varying lengths of time during the provision of care at the patient's home. This exposes the car to outside elements, which may vary outside the temperature ranges for medical products. The health care worker needs to carry limited quantities of medical products in the vehicle and check the integrity of the products prior to use. Medical products should also be brought inside the health care worker's home for storage rather than left in the car after work hours or overnight.

10.3.2. Nurse's Bag

The nurse's bag is the mobile supply container that provides the necessary equipment and supplies for the delivery of care for the patient. The bag may be made of material such as cloth or leather. The nurse's bag is carried from the nurse's car to every patient's home and has the opportunity to transmit organisms from one environment to the next. Bakunas-Kenneley et al. (2009) reported positive cultures of human pathogens on the outside of 83.6 % of nurse's bags ($n = 126$) with 15.9% positive for multidrug-resistant organisms (MDROs). In addition, positive human pathogen cultures were found on the inside of nurse's bags, with 48.4% and 6.3% positive for MDROs. The study also suggests that the more porous the material of the nurse's bag, the more likely pathogens would be found. Kenneley (2007) promotes hand hygiene for 15 seconds prior to handling equipment inside the nurse's bag and after patient contact before returning any items into the nurse's bag.

10.3.3. Equipment

The home health care provider supplies medical equipment to the patient for use in their home. Whenever the patient no longer needs the equipment, the home care provider collects it up from the patient's home and brings it back to the home care facility. The medical equipment poses a risk of microorganism transmission and needs to be covered until brought back to the facility and disinfected appropriately. Separate clean utility and dirty utility areas are necessary at the home care facility to reduce the potential of infection transmission.

10.4. MULTIDRUG-RESISTANT ORGANISMS

Mrs. Gonzalez is also diagnosed with Type II diabetes and uses Insulin to control her blood glucose. She is required to check her blood glucose before meals. A foley urinary catheter was inserted post operatively because of urinary retention and is to remain for bladder training. Mrs. Gonzalez has incidents of stool incontinence. During her hospitalization, Juanita was found to have multidrug resistant organisms (MDRO) including methicillin-resistant *Staphylococcus aureus* (MRSA).

Multidrug-resistant organisms include methicillin-resistant *Staphylococcus aureus* (MRSA), vancomycin-resistant enterococci (VRE), and certain gram-negative bacilli (Talaro and Chess, 2012). Currently, there are no data reports of clients infected or colonized with an MDRO in the home care setting. However, clients can be transferred from other settings with MDROs. Therefore, home care providers need to understand the epidemiology, risks and potential for their transmission. Whenever a home care client is transferred to a health care facility, the staff of the facility should be informed of the MDRO status (McGoldrick and Rhinehart, 2007). Dedicated equipment and supplies should be left in the patient's home to reduce the risk of infection transmission. Pets need to be restricted to reduce the possibility of being a carrier. Other special instructions, including the cleaning of household surfaces, need to be addressed (HICPAC, 2007; Kenneley, 2007).

10.5. INTERPRETATION/APPLICATION OF INFECTION CONTROL DATA

During lunch, Pamela receives notification from Southern Medical Center, a regional acute care facility, that Juanita Gonzalez is being discharged home this afternoon. The care coordinator informs Pamela that Mrs. Gonzalez is a 58 year-old female, who is being discharged from the hospital following post-operative abdominal surgery related to cancer. She contracted a health care associated infection post operatively and was started on an antibiotic regimen with a peripherally inserted central catheter (PICC). She was also placed on parenteral nutrition with a central venous catheter to allow bowel rest and provide caloric intake. Mrs. Gonzalez has a secondary diagnosis of Type II diabetes and uses Insulin to control her blood glucose.

She is required to check her blood glucose before meals. A foley urinary catheter was inserted post operatively because of urinary retention and is to remain for bladder training. Mrs. Gonzalez has incidents of stool incontinence. . . . Since Mrs. Gonzalez receives intermittent home care nursing visits and not around the clock nursing care, she and her family are responsible for maintenance of her care. Pamela begins patient and family education of the plan of care at home.

Home health care is an uncontrolled and unstructured health care setting. More times than not, assessment of the home is not done until the patient is home. The home health care nurse is independent of onsite resources and must use ingenuity and health care guidelines to guide critical thinking interventions. Knowledge and application of infection prevention and control principles are critical to reduce the risk of infection transmission.

10.6. DISCUSSION ABOUT PATIENT SAFETY AND HEALTH SYSTEM ISSUES RELATED TO ICP

Home health care providers accept patients from multiple health care settings and facilities. Each health care facility has its own policies and procedures and dedicated medical equipment. Home health care providers must be fluent in the care and maintenance of several different medical devices and physician protocols. Home health care nurses are charged with providing care to patients in their own environments and the nurse must be respectful not to intrude into the private space, nor judge the condition of the home. The aim of the nurse is to provide optimal care in a safe and clean environment. The home health nurse requires environmental flexibility to be able to transform a home setting into a viable health care area.

Home health care organizations must communicate and coordinate with other health care organizations to provide care for their clients. Rarely do patients initiate health care in their homes. As a result, home care organizations most always receive patients from other health care organizations. Communication is essential in order to be informed of the patient's health care status including infections, risks associated with infections such as indwelling invasive devices, MRDO status and vulnerability status. This information enables the health care organization to prepare and provide the best service for the client. Time is an essential component within home health care. Having the knowledge of what patient care is needed gives the home care organization the ability to allocate the personnel and time frame to conduct a safe and effective visit by having the necessary supplies for infection prevention and control. When the nurse has enough time to provide care for the patient, it is more likely that correct procedures and guidelines will be followed. Compromised practice can result in poor practices such as not taking the time for hand washing or hand hygiene (Felemban *et al.*, 2012).

Education is the cornerstone of home health care. The family and patient incur much of the responsibility of caring for the patient. They must have the necessary knowledge and willingness to comply with hand washing, transmission of infection and standards precautions. Patients and caregivers must be informed of the specific mode of transmission related to their infection. There are certain circumstances when standard precautions are not sufficient and more protection is needed (Kenneley, 2007).

Home care nursing is an autonomous practice. There is not the accessible of health care workers and resources at the bedside of the patient. There is a strong reliance on the patient and family as well as the nurses who provide the teaching and visits. Each nurse must be competent and compliant with infection prevention and control principles and reinforce and review these principles with the patient and family on each visit.

Health care associated infections are a major issue in health care organizations, and home health care is no exception. Patient safety initiatives to reduce transmission of infections are vital. Home healthcare organizations often do not have prepared infection control professionals. Surveillance is necessary to track and evaluate infection transmission in home healthcare delivery systems. Besides focusing on the reduction of transmission in the home care setting, home care surveillance may be able to provide data of those patients who develop health care associated infections and the organizations from which they received their original care. Mandatory reporting of healthcare associated infections are the trend and many states have already enacted this legislation. The time has arrived for home healthcare organizations to actively participate in the coordinated effort to reduce transmission of infections.

10.7. SUMMARY POINTS

• Home care is an uncontrolled environment that requires a

systematic evaluation and strategy to reduce the risk for transmission of infectious disease.

- The health care nurse must use his/her own hand hygiene products for hand soap and paper towels and teach patient and family/ caregivers to be vigilant in hand hygiene practices when caring for the patient to avoid transmission of infectious agents.
- Disinfection in the home environment is a significant intervention to prevent transmission of infection.
- Standard precautions may not be enough and patients need to be informed of special infections that require more protection and what additional interventions need to be employed.
- Surveillance of home care infections needs to take on a more active role.

10.8. REFERENCES

Bakunas-Kenneley, I., and Madigan, E. (2009). Infection prevention and control in home health care: The nurse's bag. *American Journal of Infection Control, 37*(8): 687–688.

Belkin, N.L. (2001). Home laundering of soiled surgical scrubs: surgical site infections and the home environment. *American Journal of Infection Control,* (29)1: 58–64.

Clark, P. (2010). Emergence of infection control surveillance in alternate health care settings. *Journal of Infusion Nursing, 33*(6): 363–378.

Cozad, A. and Jones, R.D. (2003). Disinfection and the prevention of infectious disease. *American Journal of Infection Control, 31*(4): 243–254.

Felemban. O., John, W.S., et al. (2012). Hand hygiene practices of home visiting community nurses: perceptions, compliance, techniques, and contextual factors of practice using the World Health Organization's "Five Moments for Hand Hygiene". *Home Healthcare Nurse, 30*(3): 152–60.

Jurkovich, P. (2004). Home-versus hospital-laundered scrubs: a pilot study. *The American Journal of Maternal-Child Nursing. 29*(2): 106–111.

Kenneley, I. (2007). Infection control and prevention in home healthcare: prevention activities are the key to desired patient outcomes. *Home Healthcare Nurse, 25*(7): 459–469.

Kenneley, I. (2012). Infection control in home healthcare: an exploratory study of issues for patients and providers. *Home Healthcare Nurse, 30*(4): 235–245.

Leiss, J.K., Siteman, K.L. and Kendra, M.A. (2011). Provision and use of PPE among home care and hospice nurses in North Carolina. *American Journal of Infection Control, 39*(2): 123–128.

Manangan L.P., Pearson, M.L., Tokars, J.I., Miller, E. and Jarvis, W.R. (2002). Feasibility of national surveillance of home care associated infections in homecare settings. *Emerging Infectious Diseases, 8*(3): 233–236.

McGoldrick, M. (2009). Cleaning and disinfection of patient care equipment used in the home setting. *Caring, 28*(3): 34–39.

McGoldrick, M. (2010). Preventing infections in patients using respiratory therapy equipment in the home. *Home Healthcare Nurse: The Journal for the Home Care and Hospice Professional,* 28(4): 212–20.

McGoldrick, M. and Rhinehart, E. (2007). Managing multidrug-resistant organisms in home care and hospice: surveillance, prevention and control. *Home Healthcare Nurse: The Journal for the Home Care and Hospice Professional,* 25(9): 580–6.

Talaro, K. P. and Chess, P. (2012). *Foundations in Microbiology,* 8th ed. New York: McGraw Hill.

Wiener-Well, Y., Gaulty, M., Rudensky, B., Schlesinger, Y., Attias, D. and Yinnon, A. (2011). Nursing and physican attire as possible source of nosocomial infections. *American Journal of Infection Control,* 39(7): 555–59.

CHAPTER 11

Infection Control Practice in Mental Health Settings

JAMES WEIDEL Ph.D., MSN, FNP

The case study used for this chapter will emphasize the difficulties associated with prevention of infection among mentally challenged individuals. Topics may include the transmission of communicable diseases, healthcare provider exposure to infected patients with hepatitis or HIV/ AIDS, and MRSA. Strategies as to how to provide safe patient care while adhering to the principles of infection control will be presented.

11.1. CASE PRESENTATION

Trulia Myers is a nurse practitioner who recently was hired in a psychiatric/mental health facility that is part of a larger urban medical center. She has many years of nursing experience in both acute care and psychiatric mental health settings. Recently, Trulia and her team comprised of psychiatrists, social workers, and counselors were faced with a high number of patients who were stricken with diarrheal illnesses. This outbreak was not limited to a single unit, but impacted several, including geriatric, adult, adolescent, and pediatric treatment units. Affected were a number of patients in the day treatment program and four staff nurses. The costs to the facility related to the number of lost work days for employees, paid overtime for staff covering for sick employees, longer lengths of stay, increased treatment costs, and overall inconvenience contributed to an already dire situation. This event and a number of similar smaller episodes over the past three years drew the attention of the hospital administration.

Because Trulia had experience with infection control teams in an acute care hospital, administrators requested that Trulia lead a team of staff to survey infection control practices, investigate possible sources of infection, and identify shortcomings in infection control and surveillance. She knew this would be a challenge owing to multiple differences from the acute care setting, including patients, providers, diagnoses and treatment plans, and the overall layout of the facility.

To get a general idea of how infection control practices were being conducted, Trulia and the project team decided to conduct general surveys or "walkarounds" on units to identify factors that might have been associated with the diarrhea outbreak. Trulia noticed alcohol-based hand sanitizer was only available in locked sections of the units where only nursing staff had access. There were no sinks available for patient hand washing other than in the patients' rooms, and they had no soap. Patients were routinely issued a small bar of soap or small bottle of baby shampoo in the morning for self care. However, she noticed that patients did not use all of the soap or, to save money, stockpiled the items to bring home. Even so, if patients had soap at their sinks, it still required them to walk quite a distance from group activities, day rooms, and kitchenettes to their rooms to wash their hands. Trulia and the project team suspected that some of the patients might have washed their hands only once a day during their morning routine.

Trulia and the team also made note of the laundry facilities. The laundry room was at the far end of each psychiatric unit. The facility was locked throughout the day and was available for patients to do their laundry from 7 PM to 9 PM, if staff were available. There is one washer and one dryer on a unit. The laundry detergent was kept in a locked closet and staff had to be present when the laundry door was open. Ancillary staff normally assisted with the laundry, but did not directly instruct or supervise patients laundering clothes. Because of the demands on staff to monitor patient whereabouts and activities, Trulia wondered if the laundry facilities were actually available during designated hours and if patients were being adequately instructed and supervised on how to do their laundry. She also wondered who determines when clothes need laundering—staff or patients. One team member noted laundry hours coincided with the unit's hours for television and evening hygiene. Additionally, a patient on the unit commented that she was reluctant to do laundry out of fear someone might steal her clothes.

After visiting each psychiatric unit, Trulia not only began to think about how staff nurses, mental health counselors, and patients ought to change how they approach infection control in the psychiatric setting, but she also thought about her own practice. Nurse practitioners and psychiatrists must not focus solely on mental health, but should consider preventing infection between and among patients. Trulia reflected on how she and other health care providers could do a better job during patient intake, assessment, admitting, and patient rounds to reduce the spread of infection on the units.

Since the outbreak on the unit was gastrointestinal in nature and a number of employees were affected, the team decided that it would be a good idea to visit the food service areas in the facility. Although culinary services are inspected routinely by county food inspectors and then given a grade, Trulia and the team were aware that inspectors would not investigate outbreaks of illness in a mental health facility unless complaints were filed or requests were made to the county. Before rounding in areas where food was prepared, cooked, and served, the team discussed the relevance of the inspection to employee and patient health.

After surveying the kitchens and other places where food was served and consumed, many deficient practices came to the team's attention. Trulia noted wrapped frozen chicken without labels thawing on a cutting board. In the delivery and receiving area, she noticed a service door that was open to the loading dock, allowing flies to enter. She also noticed that prepackaged snacks were provided on each unit. Not all items were wrapped. Patients took peanut butter from a large jar for sandwiches and not from individually packaged servings. A loaf of sliced bread was in a plastic bag and pizza slices uncovered and lying out on a large tray. Utensils were provided but patients commonly took items with bare hands. It was apparent that consumption of snacks was not limited to the dining area. Often a patient on the unit would take on a leadership role and prepare and distribute snacks throughout the unit. Little concern was given to personal hygiene or whether the patient washed his/her hands prior to distributing snacks. Food wrappers and snacks could be seen in patient rooms and the TV lounge area. Also, employees and patients would eat together on occasion to celebrate a birthday or a holiday. This practice was encouraged to remove perceived barriers between patients and staff and to promote a therapeutic milieu.

Trulia and the team also noticed other things that were concerning. The tables appeared to be stained with food and utensils were lying about on tables and countertops. There was a large amount of crumbs and food particles on the floor where patients prepared and consumed the food. The floor in the general area near the pantry, day room leading to patient rooms was wet and sticky from spilled coffee and juice.

Trulia Myers and the team decided to have a meeting to discuss existing infection control protocols at the facility. When they evaluated the infection control manual, they were surprised to discover the infection control manual used was intended for general medical centers. No specific recommendations were in place for psychiatric facilities. In the manual, there was frequent mention of isolation, negative pressure rooms, and personal protective equipment such as gowns, but Trulia and the other team members had not come across their use during the survey. As the team read through the medical center's general infection control protocol manual, they discussed what elements of infection control principles applied to their clinical setting. With infection control principles in mind, the team discussed the specific items unique to their setting as well as new procedures and practices that could be adopted and added to the manual. In addition, they discussed how they could educate patients and staff for the purpose of improving infection control practices in the psychiatric facility.

11.2. ENVIRONMENT OF CARE OF THE PSYCHIATRIC/MENTAL HEALTH FACILITY

Psychiatric and mental health care facilities are a heterogeneous group of institutions that provide a diverse and broad range of psychiatric, behavioral and mental health services to individuals and families (Nicolle, 2000). The behavioral impact of psychiatric patients' underlying disease alone can make infection control particularly challenging. If one takes into account the vast array of treatment settings and modalities utilized while caring for psychiatric patients, then the prevention, control, and management of outbreaks of communicable disease in psychiatric settings is no ordinary undertaking (Cheng *et al.*, 2007).

The environment in which psychiatric patients receive care differs markedly from traditional medical surgical facilities. The integration of patient and staff safety with design of the physical environment of psychiatric and behavioral health facilities requires careful consideration, extensive planning, and expertise. The main goals in the construction and design of most psychiatric facilities is to maximize patient safety, to prevent the concealment of contraband, to allow for patient privacy, and to facilitate patient care—not to minimize the transmission of disease. The unique design of psychiatric and mental health units must serve the purpose of both functional work space—in which doctors, advanced practice nurses, and support staff can interact with patients in a therapeutic environment—while at the same time protecting patient privacy and ensuring patient and employee safety. Designers, engineers, and architects of psychiatric facilities must take on other challenges; they must make psychiatric facilities appear comfortable, attractive, and as residential in character as possible. Strong efforts are made to avoid an "institutional" look and meet the therapeutic needs of patients while meeting the vast array of applicable safety and security codes and regulations (Sine and Hunt, 2009). For this reason, psychiatric nurses and infection-control practitioners must be innovative in their efforts to protect the health of psychiatric patients and employees.

11.3. LIMITED ACCESS TO SUPPLIES

Trulia noticed alcohol hand sanitizer was only available in locked sections of the units where only nursing staff had access. There were no sinks available for patient hand washing other than the sinks in patients' rooms which had no soap readily nearby and available.

Developing rational infection control strategies which can be readily implemented in often complex psychiatric settings can be a challenge for even the best prepared infection control practitioners. In behavioral health units, safety and security are of primary concern. Consequently, unit designs that are specifically intended to inhibit the spread of infection on medical surgical units may be intentionally omitted to decrease risks or dangers to patients or staff. For example, strategies intended to decrease syringe diversion by patients may lead to an inadequate supply of sharp containers. Having fewer containers increases the distance as well as the time in which a nurse has a sharp in hand from the time of injection until disposal, thereby increasing risk for a needle stick to employees. Additionally, items such as soap dispensers can be easily pulled off walls and broken into sharp shards that can be used as weapons, leading to injury to self and others (Sine and Hunt, 2009), and soap reservoirs provide concealed space in which contraband can be hidden. Furthermore, patients may ingest antiseptic hand gels from dispensers because of the alcohol content. Overall, psychiatric facilities have fewer safe locations for the installation of soap dispensers and sinks because patients may require monitoring during their use, resulting in the lack of sufficient hand washing areas.

11.4. LINEN AND CLOTHING

Trulia wondered if the laundry facilities were actually available during those hours and if patients were being adequately instructed and supervised on how to do their laundry. She also wondered who determines when clothes need laundering—the staff or the patients?

Clothing and linen are strictly monitored in psychiatric settings. Patients should have an adequate supply of either clothing or linens which should be inspected initially. Although most psychiatric facilities have a laundry available for patients to wash their clothes, supplies of detergent may be restricted due to concerns over ingestion of laundry detergents. Bleach is seldom provided due to the caustic nature and danger of ingestion and because bleach may be used to color hair and clothing. Due to restricted access to laundry supplies, patients may be inclined to launder clothes without detergent or with an inadequate amount. This process may remove dirt and odors, but is inadequate for killing pathogenic organisms. Patients should be instructed on how to use the laundry facilities properly. Staff should distribute laundry detergent and provide adequate and safe supervision of its use (Bick, 2007). Routine inspections should be performed to ensure that machines, lint traps, and mechanical operation of the laundry equipment meet the manufacturer recommendations and physical safety codes.

11.5. PROVIDER-PATIENT INTERACTION

It is not only staff nurses, mental health counselors, and patients that may need to change how they approach infection control in the psychiatric setting. Nurse practitioners and psychiatrists should not solely focus on mental health, but should also consider preventing infection between and among patients. Trulia began to evaluate how she and other health care providers could do a better job during patient intake, assessment, admitting, and patient rounds to reduce the spread of infection on the units.

Outbreaks of infectious diseases in psychiatric facilities are not uncommon and yet are only occasionally reported in the literature. Most healthcare acquired infections (HAIs) on psychiatric and behavioral health units are respiratory tract infections, followed by enteric and skin infections (Cheng *et al.*, 2007). Many infections go undiagnosed or are overlooked when patients are admitted to psychiatric units. For example, skin and soft-tissue infections have often been mistakenly diagnosed as spider bites, which were in actuality infections positive for methicillin-resistant Staphylococcus aureus (MRSA). Misdiagnosis of skin infections results in delay of appropriate treatment and the possibility that unidentified infections could be spread to other patients on the unit. Many prudent infection control policies dictate that soft-tissue lesions should be considered MRSA until proven otherwise. Bearing in mind the large number of psychiatric patients who are immunocompromised or infected with HIV, delayed or missed medications and treatment places other patients at risk, lengthens duration of stay, and increases costs associated with inpatient psychiatric care (Gilbride *et al.*, 2009).

Despite little mention in peer reviewed journals and greater emphasis on infection control in medical surgical and acute care hospital settings (versus psychiatric settings), the importance of infection control in psychiatric and mental health facilities should not be underestimated. Because the focus for mental-health providers evaluating patients is on psychiatric diagnosis and treatment, providers may unwittingly fail to identify sources of infection or modes of transmission to and from patients or visitors. Such inattention may lead to delays in medical evaluation, outbreak recognition, and disease eradication.

11.6. FOOD SAFETY

Trulia and the team were aware that inspectors routinely do not investigate outbreaks of illness in a mental health facility unless complaints were filed or requests were made with the county. Before rounding in areas where food was prepared, cooked, and served, the team discussed some of their findings and relevance to employee and patient health.

Foodborne illnesses due to Noroviruses, *Campylobacter jejuni, Sal-*

monella enteritidis, Shigella, Staphylococcus, and *Streptococcus pyogenes* are commonly reported in psychiatric facilities. By preventing foodborne illnesses, foodservice personnel employed in institutional settings have an important role in protecting the health of patients and employees. Foodborne pathogens pose a threat of illness, but the risk of illness is relatively small when food is prepared and handled by food service personnel who have been trained to prepare and handle food using proper safety techniques (Puckett, 1998).

In addition to constant hand washing, all food-service employees should adhere to basic infection control guidelines regarding culinary services. Management should make serious efforts to interview and hire the appropriate persons for the job and orient staff (not just food-service workers) on principles of safe and sanitary food handling. Food-service employees in particular must be provided with measurable, competency-based job descriptions that include food-handling precautions recommended by federal and local health departments. Examples of food handling control measures to reduce risk of food-borne illnesses include freezing raw meat and poultry that will not be used within 1 to 2 days, using refrigerated ground meat and meat patties within 2 days, never thawing meat or poultry at room temperature, and refrigerating foods containing cooked meat or poultry within 2 hours after cooking. Other conventions include keeping hot foods hot [at or above 140°F (60°C)] and cold foods cold [at or below 40°F (4°C)] (Puckett, 1998). Employees should carefully follow "keep refrigerated" and "use by" labels.

Culinary work in institutions must include sanitization measures that are integrated in regular food preparation routines. Such responsibilities include completely washing all fruits (including bananas, melons, and citrus fruits) and vegetables before peeling or eating, hand washing, and maintaining the facility and equipment in sanitary and safe conditions. Other straightforward measures include providing color-coded cutting boards for meats, raw foods, and ready-to-eat foods, cleaning and sanitizing cutting boards, utensils, and surfaces after use; and avoiding cross-contamination from knives and cutting boards to food (Puckett, 1998).

In facilities with patients or residents who are highly susceptible to infection, food service managers, workers, and dietitians should make menu choices that avoid foods deemed high risk for contamination by pathogens. Examples include apples and beverages that may contain apple juice. Such products should be pasteurized or obtained in commercially sterile shelf stable form and in hermetically sealed containers.

Pasteurized shell eggs or pasteurized liquid, frozen, or dry eggs should be substituted for raw eggs in shells when preparing sauces, creams and egg-fortified beverages. Raw animal food such as raw fish, raw marinated fish, raw shellfish, or partially cooked or undercooked foods such as rare meats and soft-cooked eggs should never be served (Puckett, 1998).

Employees should not be allowed to handle food when ill (Hall *et al.*, 2011). Employees who develop an illness that can be transmitted through culinary work should be promptly unassigned until medically cleared to return. Routine inspections should be performed to ensure compliance with published standards for hand washing facilities, hygiene, and food storage temperatures. In addition, routine control measures should be in place for cleanup procedures that include washing of utensils and work areas with hot water and antibacterial cleaning agents as well as plans for pest and vermin control.

11.7. PATIENT HANDLING OF FOOD

Patients were free to take peanut butter from a larger jar, not individually packaged servings. A loaf of sliced bread was in a plastic bag and pizza slices uncovered and lying out on a large tray. Utensils were provided, but patients commonly took items with bare hands.

Bare hands should not be used when distributing ready-to-eat foods (foods edible without washing, cooking, or additional preparation to achieve food safety). This rule is recommended for all employees and patients, whether working in a culinary capacity or not. This can be achieved by using utensils such as tongs, forks, or scoops, or by wearing non-sterile food service grade gloves. Utensils should be washed in hot soapy water and dried thoroughly on a daily basis (Hall *et al.*, 2011). Patients should be discouraged from storing, preparing, and eating perishable food in their rooms. Psychiatric patients who have poorly controlled mental illness, hygiene, or lack the intellectual ability to adhere to appropriate standards of hygiene ought not to assist in handling or delivering of food. Members of infection control teams or professionals conducting surveillance should note that, when investigating an outbreak of gastrointestinal illness, it is important to consider other sources of food, including food in patients' rooms and food delivered in packages by visitors.

11.8. SANITATION AND HOUSEKEEPING

The tables appeared to be stained with food and there were utensils lying about on tables. There were large amounts of crumbs and food particles on the floor where patients prepared and consumed food. The floor in the general area near the pantry, day room, and leading to patient rooms was wet and sticky where coffee and juice had been spilled.

As with medical facilities, the role of sanitation and housekeeping staff in maintaining a clean and safe environment is important. For example, hospitals that report lower rates of *Clostridium difficile* infection also report higher infection surveillance and greater scores of cleanliness of patient areas (Hannon-Engel and Fantasia, 2010). Despite this, considerable variation exists with regard to cleaning and disinfecting protocols in hospitals (Wilkinson *et al.*, 2011). Psychiatric facilities should be made easy to clean and maintain. Water, mops, brooms, detergents, and cleansers should be easily accessible to employees, but completely inaccessible to patients. Beyond straightforward and routine cleaning, janitorial services or housekeeping should maintain a regimen detailing features such as doorframes, casework, and finish transitions to avoid dirt-catching and hard-to-clean crevices and joints (Tseng *et al.*, 2011). Additionally, housekeeping should maintain chemicals and supplies either off the unit or on the unit within a durable locking cabinet in a locked closet or nurses' station. Frequent inspections by housekeeping departments along with nursing staff should be conducted (Bick, 2007). Procedures should be in place to allow adequate time for janitorial services to complete the assigned housekeeping tasks. Coordination with the therapeutic use of space on the mental health units is important. Often housekeeping may be reluctant to clean areas when patients occupy a room or where group therapy is occurring. Cleaning schedules should be coordinated with patient care activities to ensure cleaning is completed and housekeeping staff feel comfortable and confident performing their jobs.

11.9. RISK FACTORS ASSOCIATED WITH INFECTION AMONG PSYCHIATRIC PATIENTS

Patients who receive psychiatric and mental health services range from pediatric to geriatric. Patients may be admitted of their own volition, by family members, the police, the courts, or may be admitted from medical surgical units for psychiatric care. Psychiatric patients are unique in the sense that they may have a number of limitations that put them at risk for HAIs. Mental illness often complicates the appropriate management of contagious illnesses. Patients are institutionalized because they have significant issues with mental health and impaired functional status, thereby increasing their risk for colonization with resistant organisms (Nicolle, 2000; Muder, 1998). Sometimes violent behavior on psychiatric units makes infection control measures difficult to implement.

Psychiatric patients also suffer from poor nutrition and other comorbidities associated with risk of infection or colonization with resistant organisms. For example, institutionalized psychiatric patients are at higher risk for MRSA due to prolonged hospitalization, skin lacerations and abrasions, previous antibiotic use, poor hygiene, performing their own wound care, inadequate laundering of clothes, and lack of access to care. Compared with general patients, psychiatric patients have an increased prevalence of HIV, hepatitis B and C viruses, syphilis, gonorrhea, chlamydia, and tuberculosis. Ectoparasites, such as scabies and lice, are common problems among institutional psychiatric patient populations (Bick, 2007), yet early recognition of index cases is commonly missed (Nicolle, Garibaldi and Strausbaugh, 1996). A clinician should promptly evaluate all patients who have pruritus, rashes, or skin lesions. Appropriate management of suspected cases includes oral and topical medication, clothing and linen exchange, and laundering.

In addition to pathogens commonly transmitted by respiratory and fecal-oral routes, employees are exposed to blood-borne pathogens during medical, housekeeping and laundry duties. Syringes, tattoo paraphernalia, and weapons may be encountered during inspection of clothes and personal belongings, especially during admission. Nurses commonly administer intramuscular injections to patients who are agitated or combative, which puts nurses at risk for accidental needle sticks. Employees may also be exposed to spitting, throwing of body fluids, and fecal smearing by patients. Staff should be vigilant and wear clean non-sterile gloves when at risk of touching blood, body fluids, secretions, excretions, contaminated items, mucous membranes, and non-intact skin. Gloves should be changed between procedures on the same patient and between patients. Providers should perform hand-hygiene immediately after a procedure.

Infection control practices in psychiatric settings are particularly challenging, as hand hygiene protocols are more specific to acute care facilities (Cheng *et al.*, 2007). Because access to soap and water and ethanol-based hand sanitizers is limited due to safety concerns, scheduled hand hygiene times should be implemented. Traditional methods of teaching proper hand washing and other infection control techniques may not apply to psychiatric patients, so staff may need to assist patients with hand hygiene. Staff should witness or assist patients washing or cleansing their hands prior to exiting their rooms in the morning. Scheduled times should include prior to all meals and snacks upon returning from smoking breaks, and after playing with cards, board games, or whenever hands are visibly soiled (Cheng *et al.*; Gilbride *et al.*, 2009). Staff should account for possible contraband like soap and sanitizer.

11.10. ISOLATION

In the manual, there was frequent mention of isolation, negative pressure rooms, and personal protective equipment like gowns, but Trulia and the other team members had not come across their use during the survey.

Patients in psychiatric care facilities are highly vulnerable to infection, and their mobility increases the opportunity for disease transmission. The unique nature in the way care is delivered may explain the rapid spread of infection in patients or staff in mental health facilities. The need for frequent group activities for therapy (Tseng *et al.*, 2011) means that a greater portion of the environment is dedicated to communal space in locked units, thereby facilitating greater interaction between staff and increased patient-to-patient contact. Frequent crowding and rationed access to soap, water, and clean laundry also increases the probability of transmission of potentiality pathogenic organisms and contributes to the high attack rates when infections do occur. Moreover, the abrupt pattern of admission and discharge—typical of mental health institutions—also complicates the diagnosis of infection.

There are several differences when characterizing infection control programs between acute medical surgical units and psychiatric facilities (Cheng *et al.*, 2007). Infection control measures in psychiatric facilities are often ignored because these facilities have fewer resources in terms of personnel, clinical experience, and diagnostic services to implement infection control protocols compared to medical care facilities (Nicolle, 2000). Persons responsible for infection control usually have multiple responsibilities and may not have a level of training equivalent to that of practitioners in acute care facilities. In addition, infection control supplies are commonly lacking due to budget concerns and perceptions that they are not needed in the unique setting. Examples include the lack of specialized isolation rooms and personal protective equipment (Gilbride *et al.*, 2009). Psychiatric institutions which do have personal protective equipment may limit access to the equipment because, like many other items, locking the items discourages theft. The extra steps and effort may discourage health care workers from taking the time to don necessary personal protective equipment. As a result, staff may ignore or downplay its use, consequently putting both staff and patients at risk for transmissible pathogens.

11.11. TRANSMISSION BASED PRECAUTIONS

As the team read through the medical center's general infection control protocol manual, they discussed what elements of infection control principles also applied to their clinical setting.

Considering the highly infectious nature of HAIs, exclusion and isolation of infected persons is often the most practical means of interrupting disease transmission and limiting contamination of the environment. Exclusion and isolation is particularly important in settings where people reside or congregate, such as residential or domiciliary style treatment facilities. Because empirical evidence for the effectiveness of exclusion and isolation strategies is limited, strategies for transmission and infection control should be based on common infection-control principles. The principle underpinning isolation is to minimize contact with persons during the most infectious periods of their illness and, in some cases, exclusion of exposed and potentially incubating persons (Hall *et al.*, 2011).

Isolation of both exposed and unexposed well persons might be useful during outbreaks in psychiatric facilities to help break the chain of infection and prevent additional cases. In healthcare facilities, ill patients may be cohorted together in a unit, or part thereof, with dedicated nursing staff to provide care for infected persons. However, in psychiatric settings many patients cannot be in "like" rooms because of behavior disorders or aggression.

Outbreak detection and transmission control in the psychiatric setting is often complicated by the inability to confine a source patient to his or her room. In the psychiatric setting, patients under droplet precautions should be assigned to private rooms. When patients cannot be accommodated in single occupancy rooms, efforts should be made to separate them from asymptomatic patients. All non-cohorted individuals must wear masks within 3 feet of individuals on precautions. Considerations should be made to restrict symptomatic and recovering patients from leaving patient-care areas unless it is essential for treatment. Overall attempts should be made to minimize patient movements within a ward (MacCannell *et al.*, 2011). This may involve suspending group activities for the duration of an outbreak or closing wards to new admissions or transfers as a measure to attenuate the magnitude of an outbreak.

Dependent upon facility characteristics, approaches for cohorting patients during outbreaks may include placing patients in multi-occupancy rooms or contiguous sections within a facility for patient cohorts (Hall *et al.*, 2011). Staff should restrict symptomatic and recovering patients from leaving patient-care areas unless it is essential for treatment. Longer periods of isolation or cohorting precautions should be considered for complex medical patients (e.g., those with cardiovascular, autoimmune, immunosuppressive, or renal disorders), as their recovery may be prolonged (MacCannell *et al.*, 2011). Vigilance and strict adherence to hand hygiene among healthcare personnel, patients, and visitors in patient care should be enforced.

11.12. RESTRAINTS AND INFECTION CONTROL

Considering effective and feasible infection control principles, the team discussed specific practices that were unique to their work setting that could be added or adapted to their infection control manual. They also discussed how they could educate patients and staff to improve infection control practices in the psychiatric facility.

When restraints and protective devices are used, they should be cleaned and stored between uses in accordance with the manufacturer's recommended guidelines. In the absence of guidelines, sensible infection control principles apply and should be followed. Items like Posey wrist restraints and Posey vests should be washed using an approved disinfectant cleaner and rinsed and dried completely. When dry, the device should be stored in a closed plastic bag that is clearly labeled with the cleaning date. Leather restraints should be wiped clean after each use, using an approved disinfectant cleaner, and then rinsed with water and allowed to air dry for at least 30 minutes. When dry, a commercially made leather cleaner and conditioner should be applied and the leather should be allowed to dry for at least one hour. The leather restraints should then be placed in a plastic container with the cleaning date.

Published guidelines for the diagnosis and treatment of communicable diseases are not readily applicable to psychiatric institutions. Nonetheless, opportunities exist for infectious disease specialists and infection control practitioners to have an impact on psychiatric patients and the communities in which they live. Infection control education should be provided at the initiation of employment and regularly thereafter (Hannon-Engel and Fantasia, 2010). Effective implementation of infection control programs should limit the occurrence and extent of outbreaks. Although limited laboratory testing is the norm in psychiatric settings, criteria for when to obtain laboratory specimens should be clearly delineated. Criteria will vary based on institutional characteristics and resources, but should include prompt identification of potential clusters for respiratory illnesses, gastroenteritis, and skin infections (Nicolle, 2000).

Training should include all staff—especially those providing direct care to patients (Freeman, 2011). All education programs should be documented with the names of attendees, date, topic and evaluations. Programs should be timely and reflect the current state of knowledge regarding pathogenesis, transmission, and prevention. Basic hygiene, hand hygiene, transmission of diseases, employee health, prevention and susceptibility of diseases should be included. Surveillance data appropriate to improve staff compliance with infection control practices may be included during education sessions (Smith and Rusnak, 1997). Compliance not only requires education of all staff, but also an evaluation of the program for effectiveness (Hannon-Engel and Fantasia, 2010).

Every psychiatric facility should have a written exposure control plan that includes vaccination of at-risk staff, education of the use of personal protective equipment, environmental controls to decrease the likelihood of sharps injuries, and a post exposure prophylaxis program. Prompt follow-up evaluation of exposed employees must be ensured. To reduce delay in treatment, clinicians at psychiatric facilities should be authorized to initiate post-exposure prophylaxis for employees. A post-exposure control plan in psychiatric facilities should also provide non-occupational post-exposure prophylaxis to patients who experience a significant potential exposure to pathogens, which may include blood-borne pathogens.

11.13. CONCLUSION

Psychiatric and mental health facilities are a unique set of institutions that specifically serve patients with mental health and behavioral problems. The environment in which patients receive care differs greatly from that of traditional medical and surgical healthcare delivery systems. Despite the lesser amount of emphasis on infection control, HAIs within the mental health setting do commonly occur. All employees including healthcare professionals, administrative, clerical, janitorial, and food service workers must work together to reduce the risk of HAIs. Comprehensive plans and protocols that take into account sound infection-control principles within the context of a mental-healthcare delivery system must be developed to ensure safety. Plans for infection control should include employee education and training, monitoring of strict compliance, and periodic review of, and modifications to, infection control manuals, guidelines, and protocols. Because of the unique nature of the psychiatric setting, special attention must be paid to patients' and employees' physical safety and risk for exposure to disease causing pathogens. Plans for infection control must include common sources of HAIs such as food-borne diarrheal illnesses and ways in which sanitation, personal hygiene, hand-washing, housekeeping, and food preparation duties can be performed to ensure a safe working environment to employees and safe delivery of quality care to their patients.

11.14. SUMMARY POINTS

- Safety and security of patients include infection control
- Respiratory, enteric and skin infections are most common in mental health facilities
- Large numbers of mental health patients may be immunocompromised
- Food handling should be carefully monitored due to multiple staff and patient involvement in the preparation and distribution of food
- Laundering may need to be taught or monitored closely when facilities are available for patient use

- Cleaning supplies should be easily accessible to staff, but completely unavailable to patients
- Infection control policies should not be ignored when caring for combatitive or violent patients
- All skin lesions should be assessed by a clinician since MRSA and parasitic infestations are common in this population
- Scheduled hand hygiene may be needed
- Patient mobility may accelerate the spread of infectious diseases

11.15. REFERENCES

Bick, J.A. (2007). Infection control in jails and prisons. *Clinical Infectious Diseases, 45*: 1047–1055.

Cheng, V.C., Wu, A.L., Cheung, C.Y., *et al.* (2007). Outbreak of human metapneumovirus infection in psychiatric inpatients: Implications for directly observed use of lcohol hand rub in prevention of nosocomial infections. *Journal of Hospital Infection, 67*: 336–343. doi:10.1016/j.jhin.2007.09.010

Freeman, S. (2011). Charge nurses' perceptions of infection control. *Mental Health Practice, 14*: 26–29.

Gilbride, S.J., Lee, B.E., Taylor, G.D. and Forgie, S.E. (2009). Successful containment of a norovirus outbreak in an acute adult psychiatric area. *Infection Control and Hospital Epidemiology, 30*: 289–291.

Gould, D. (2008). Management and prevention of norovirus outbreaks in hospitals. *Nursing Standard, 23*: 51–56.

Hall, A.J., Vinje, J., Lopman, B., Park, G.W., *et al.* (2011). Updates to norovirus outbreak management and disease prevention guidelines. *MMWR, 60*(3): 1–15.

Hannon-Engel, S. and Fantasia, H.C. (2010). Are you ready? Online evaluation of a multi-drug resistant organisms education program in a behavioral health hospital. *Perspectives in Psychiatric Care, 47*: 138–144.

Maccannell, T., Umscheid, C.A., Agarwal, R.K., Lee, I., Kuntz, G., Stevenson, K.B. and Healthcare Infection Control Practices Advisory Committee (2011). Guideline for the prevention and control of norovirus gastroenteritis outbreaks in healthcare settings. *Infection Control and Hospital Epidemiology, 32*: 939–969. doi:10.1086/662025

Muder, R.R. (1998). Pneumonia in residents of long-term care facilities: Epidemiology, etiology, management, and prevention. *American Journal of Medicine, 105*: 319–330.

Nicolle, L.E. (2000). Infection control in long-term care facilities. *Clinical Infectious Diseases, 31*: 752–756.

Nicolle, L.E., Garibaldi, R. and Strausbaugh, L., J. (1996). Infections and antibiotic resistance in nursing home. *Clinical Microbiological Reviews, 9*: 1–17.

Puckett, R.P. (1998). Food safety in long-term care facilities. *Topics in Clinical Nutrition, 14*: 16–25.

Sine, D.M. and Hunt, J.M. (2009). Design Guide for the Built Environment of Behavioral Health Facilities (Edition 3.0). Washington DC: National Association of Psychiatric Health Systems.

Smith, P.W. and Rusnak, P.G. (1997). Infection prevention and control in the long-term care facility. *Infection Control and Hospital Epidemiology, 18*: 831–849.

Tseng, C.Y., Chen, C.H., Su, F.T., *et al.* (2011). Characteristics of norovirus gastroenteritis outbreaks in a psychiatric center. *Epidemiology and Infection, 139*: 275–285. doi:10.1017/S0950268810000634

Wilkinson, K., Gravel, D., Taylor, G., *et al.* (2011). Infection prevention and control practices related to Clostridium difficile infection in Canadian acute and long-term institutions. *American Journal of Infection Control, 39*: 177–182. doi:10.1016/ajic.2011.01.007

CHAPTER 12

Infection Control in Ambulatory Surgical Centers

JUDITH SELTZER, RN, MS, CNOR

The focus of this chapter will begin with a patient safety issue about an infection acquired at an ambulatory surgical center. The basic concepts associated with the infection control principles that are regulated and those that are not will be discussed. The major issues surrounding how an advanced practice healthcare provider would prevent the transmission of infection from patient to patient will be discussed. Additional topics will include disinfection, instrumentation, sterilization, healthcare worker and patient safety.

12.1. CASE PRESENTATION

Ann has been an Operating Room Nurse for over 20 years and every time a family member has to have surgery, she is the first who is called. During the weekend, Ann's mother phoned to tell her that her aunt was having surgery the following week at the Ambulatory Surgery Center near her parent's home. Although she keeps up with current regulations, Ann decided to review the recommended guidelines associated with Ambulatory Surgery Centers. She discovered that there were recently revised guidelines from the Centers for Medicare and Medicaid as well as new Recommended Practices from the Association of periOperative Registered Nurses.

During her phone conversation with her mother, Ann discovered that her aunt continued to have numbness and weakness in her left hand and will be undergoing a surgical procedure known as "left carpal tunnel release". Ann's mother asked her to explain the procedure which Ann does without hesitation. When they are finished with their phone call, Ann is reassured that her mother is satisfied and feeling better about the information shared. However, Ann is not so assured herself.

189

During their call, Ann asked her mother why the surgery was scheduled at the surgery center and not the hospital. Her mother's reply did not reassure her since she feels that the surgery center is not the right place for her aunt's surgery. Over the past 12 months, selective outpatient procedures had been moved to the surgery center location since the surgical center is affiliated with the hospital. Her aunt's surgeon operates at both locations but all procedures of this nature have been scheduled at the surgery center to free up more operating room time in the main operating room (OR) at the hospital.

Ann's mother called back later that evening and felt it was important for Ann to review her aunt's preoperative instructions. Ann assured her mother that she would review the preoperative instructions and give her aunt a call after she did so. Her aunt brought Ann the preoperative information packet and as Ann reviewed the information she was surprised to see there were no clear guidelines related to preoperative bathing before the surgical procedure.

This caused Ann much concern since she knows that all surgical patients should receive preoperative bathing instructions prior to their operative procedure. As she discussed this with her mother and aunt, both were confused, since last year her mother was instructed to initiate preoperative bathing prior to her back surgery which was performed at the hospital. Her mother asked Ann if this was normal and if the hospital and surgical center had different guidelines for surgery based on where the surgical procedure was performed. Ann was able to reinforce her knowledge after she reviewed the current AORN Recommended Practices for Hand Hygiene and Skin Antisepsis. Additionally, Ann reviewed the 1999 Center for Disease Control and Prevention statement that recommends requiring patients to shower or bathe with an antiseptic agent at least the night before or morning of the operative day (Category B-identified as being strongly recommended, based on some scientific evidence).

In this case, Ann decided to review the new Medicare's Condition for Coverage. In addition, she also decided to review the AORN's RP for Skin Antisepsis. Although she knew that all patients having surgery in her facility were instructed to take two CHG showers, she wanted to be sure that this same plan of care applied to the ASC facility. By doing so, Ann thought that she would be more prepared to discuss any infection control questions with staff at the ambulatory surgery center. During her aunt's preoperative planning appointment, Ann asked the nurse if her aunt would be instructed to take a preoperative shower with CHG the night before and morning of surgery. The nurse confirmed that general body cleansing with 4% CHG was the standard of care at the ASC and instructions were usually given during the preoperative planning visit. The nurse reviewed the bathing instructions with Ann and her aunt. When they left the facility, Ann was confident that safe infection control strategies would be followed at the ASC and her aunt will be discharged without the risk of infection.

12.2. ESSENTIAL CONTENT FOR INFECTION CONTROL IN AMBULATORY SURGICAL SETTINGS

During their call, Ann asked her mother why the surgery was scheduled at the surgery center and not the hospital.

The practice of health care is changing. The drive for expansion of services and overwhelming initiatives to reduce financial costs has provided opportunities for surgical procedures to be performed in free standing ambulatory surgery centers (ASCs). Nearly 57 million outpatient procedures are performed annually in the United States, 14 million of which occur in elderly patients. The number of ASCs has more than doubled since the 1990s, with more than 5,000 ASC facilities currently in operation nationwide (Manchikanti *et al.*, 2011). To further demonstrate the magnitude of ASC growth in the United States, CMS has identified the following 2008 statistics (US HHS, 2011):

- ASCs served 3.3 million Medicare beneficiaries
- ASCs that were Medicare certified totaled more than 5000
- ASCs that were physician owned totaled more than 300 new facilities annually

With more than 5300 ASCs opening yearly, it is easy to understand that ASCs are the fastest growing healthcare facility. With this growth, the incidence of healthcare associated infections (HAIs) becomes a priority. In 2008, a large HAI outbreak of Hepatitis C occurred in two Nevada-based ASCs as a result of poor infection control practices. The incident prompted the Center for Medicaid Services (CMS) to implement a sustained nationwide response to improve the agency's ability to detect deficient infection control practices among ASCs (Barie, 2010).

Ambulatory care settings should have the same infection prevention and control requirements as inpatient hospital settings. However, the methods used to comply with the standards vary depending on the type of care provided. The settings range from clinics that provide medical specialty expertise to clinics that perform invasive procedures, such as hemodialysis, endoscopy, and surgical centers. There are many challenges in ambulatory care to reduce infection risk and to improve patient safety. Infection control oversight and accountability is often lacking, especially if the clinics are not part of a greater hospital system. As a result of this continued growth and the increased incidence of HAIs, more emphasis must be placed on infection control practices outside of the traditional hospital facilities.

This chapter aims to discuss the current and often challenging infection prevention guidelines that are currently used in ambulatory surgery centers. Advanced practice practitioners will develop a better understanding of the evidenced-based strategies that will ensure good patient care outcomes that will improve patient and family satisfaction of their ASC facility.

12.3. REGULATORY INFLUENCES

Although she keeps up with current regulations, Ann decided to review the recommended guidelines associated with Ambulatory Surgery Centers. She discovered that there were recently revised guidelines from the Centers for Medicare and Medicaid as well as new Recommended Practices from the Association of periOperative Registered Nurses.

The revised regulations from the Centers for Medicare and Medicaid (CMS) state that all ASCs must maintain an infection control program that will minimize infections and communicable diseases. Within the standards are two guidelines that accompany this document:

A. Maintaining a sanitary environment and
B. Maintaining an infection control program.

Providers that do not comply with these guidelines will not be reimbursed for services rendered (Evans, 2009). Therefore, ASC providers must maintain compliance with infection control practices to assure a safe patient environment.

12.3.1. Standard A: Maintaining a Sanitary Environment

Since the majority of ASCs report low infection rates, some might argue that low infection rates are related to the fact that most ASCs often do not perform difficult and complex surgeries, nor do they routinely treat highly infected patients. These facts are all the more reason to maintain and comply with rigorous infection control standards. Since most patients are generally not "at-risk" for infections prior to surgery, ensuring a sanitary environment allows the patient to be free of infection resulting from their surgical procedure performed at an ASC. In fact, the Medicare revised Conditions document, 416.51, reviews many such standards with the following identified as the top five (Evans, 2009).

12.3.1.1. Standard A1: Traffic Flow

Traffic flow is not only concerned with protecting the patients' privacy but also impacts infection prevention. The ASC operating room (OR) should follow the same traffic "restrictions" as an operating room in the hospital. The association between movement through the operating room and acquisition of an infection became apparent when surgeons determined that protective clinical practices could be affected by their proximity to the patient. For example, prior to the turn of the century, surgeons wore street clothes covered by aprons into the OR. Development of surgical asepsis in the latter half of the nineteenth century was instrumental since surgeons learned that patients had fewer infections when they adopted protective surgical attire. Dr. Halsted wore a sterile gown and gloves and utilized a semicircular instrument table to separate him from observers attired in street clothes. By 1950, Operating Room restrictions and aseptic and sterile procedures were recommended and based on location (Phillips *et al.*, 2012):

The basic recommendations for OR traffic patterns consist of three major areas: *Unrestricted*—usually located near the main entrance to the OR. In this area staff, patients and vendors can dress in normal attire. *Semi-restricted*—this area represents the outer core such as the operating room suite, supply room, and instrument room. In this area, staff must wear appropriate surgical attire that includes scrub suit, disposable caps and dedicated shoes. Families are not usually permitted in this area and patients are presented in facility managed gowns with hair covered by disposable caps. If vendors, students or other visitors are present they must be dressed in appropriate surgical attire as well. *Restricted*—this area is the actual operating room, instrument room, supply room and includes the scrub sink area. In this area, appropriate surgical attire, which includes scrub suit, disposable hat, dedicated shoes or shoe covers and a mask, must be worn by all staff, students, vendors and other visitors. Patient or family members who are allowed during induction for pediatric patients should be dressed appropriately as well. ASC managers are charged with managing traffic flow for staff, patients, visitors and supplies to avoid cross contamination. With the limited space and close proximity found in ASCs, staff must avoid becoming complacent when assessing the traffic flow areas.

12.3.1.2. Standard A2: Environmental Conditions

The foundation of any ASC's sanitary environment is centered around how well the filtration system and air exchange processes work. In the hospital setting, this is usually maintained by a separate department of employees who monitor the humidity and temperature on a routine basis. In the ASC, this task must be completed on a daily basis and is often completed by the ASC manager or other designated employee. This means a good understanding of how to trouble shoot when filters need to be changed and keeping up with air flow regulations. Monitoring the ASC means monitoring air flow, humidity and temperature in the operating rooms, storage areas, decontamination area and sterile processing area.

12.3.1.3. Standard A3: Surgical Attire

In order to properly assess where and how contamination issues occur, the ASC must have a surgical attire policy implemented and understood by the staff. One of the biggest areas for concern continues to be the question of whether staff should wear scrubs brought in from home versus scrubs that are laundered by the ASC. Currently the Association of Operating Room Nurses (AORN) has recommended that practices associated with "surgical attire" should be implemented as they are in a hospital environment. It is generally accepted that healthcare workers' uniforms become contaminated with bacteria during the administration of care, particularly during surgical procedures and wound care.

Laundering of surgical attire is a global issue. How surgical attire is laundered becomes an extremely important issue to payors wanting to decrease cross contamination and HAIs. Scrub suits laundered by the facility and hair covered by a disposable cap is the recommended practice in today's surgical arena regardless of type of surgical area. Gerba (2007) reviewed a typical home-laundering process; wash cycle with detergent alone, rinse cycle and a 28-minute permanent press drying cycle. Results showed significant concentrations of Adenovirus, Rotavirus, and Hepatitis A virus had survived the home laundering process. The study further identified that these viruses could be transferred from the contaminated garments to uncontaminated garments (Gerber and Kennedy, 2007). There are nine recommended practices reviewed under AORN's recommended practices that provide additional guidance to ASC's surgical attire policy (AORN, 2011a).

12.3.1.4. Standard A4: Instrument Disinfection and Sterilization

Another fundamental aspect of a sanitary environment is that of adherence to proper cleaning and sterilization techniques. Time, temperature, pressure and type of sterilization process used must be completed according to policy and clear documentation of the process is essential. According to Medicare 416.51(a), Unwrapped/uncontained (Flash) sterilization should not be the routine but only used in an emergency for a specific device or when an instrument is accidentally dropped from the table (CMS, 2009). Flash sterilization is often seen more in the ASC environment than in the hospital environment because of the high turnover rate of patients and short procedures. However, flash sterilization should only be performed when absolutely necessary with diligent and timely documentation. Flash sterilization should not be performed simply because the number of patients scheduled is more than the amount of instrument trays that the ASC has available. Staff working in the ASC must ensure that proper and adequate training has been completed so that staff can be compliant to the recommended guidelines set forth for ASCs (CDC, 2011).

12.3.1.5. Standard A5: Facility Cleaning

Ambulatory care facilities should establish policies and procedures for routine cleaning and disinfection of environmental surfaces as part of their infection prevention plan. Key recommendations for cleaning and disinfection should include the following:

- Implement a procedure for routine cleaning that would focus on surfaces that are in close proximity to the patient and on those surfaces that are frequently touched by patients and staff alike.
- Use only EPA-registered detergents and disinfectants appropriately labeled.

- Always follow the manufacturer's recommendations and specific product instructions that will ensure product effectiveness. In addition, disposal of all items must be followed according to the regulations without exceptions (NFPA, 2005).

12.3.2. Standard B: Maintaining an Infection Control Program

Ann was able to reinforce her knowledge after she reviewed the current AORN Recommended Practices for Hand Hygiene and Skin Antisepsis.

12.3.2.1. Hand Hygiene

Hand hygiene has been identified as the single best method for reducing hand to hand pathogen transmission. When hands are visibly soiled, it is important to know that alcohol-based hand rubs should not be used exclusively in place of washing hands with either soap and water or chlorhexidine gluconate (CHG). To ensure that dispensers are installed and maintained properly, alcohol based products should be included in routine safety inspections in the ASC and should follow *NFPA 30: Flammable and Combustible Liquids Code* (Mangram *et al.*, 1999). Adherence to the Centers for Disease Control hand hygiene policies continue to be recommended for use by all healthcare personnel working in ASCs.

Ann reviewed the 1999 Center for Disease Control and Prevention statement that recommends requiring patients to shower or bathe with an antiseptic agent at least the night before or morning of the operative day (Category B-identified as being strongly recommended, based on some scientific evidence).

12.3.2.2. General Skin Cleansing

The goal of preoperative skin preparation is to:

1. reduce the risk of postoperative surgical site infection by removing loose, dead skin cells, soil and transient microorganisms from the skin;
2. reduce the resident microbial count to sub-pathogenic levels in a short period of time and with the least amount of tissue irritation;

3. Inhibit rapid, rebound growth of microorganisms (AORN, 2011a);
4. Unless contraindicated, patients should be instructed or assisted to perform two preoperative baths or showers with 4% Chlorhexidine Gluconate (CHG) before surgery to reduce the number of microorganisms on the skin and reduce the risk of subsequent contamination of the surgical wound. Following AORN's Recommended Practice on Skin Antisepsis, patients undergoing open Class I surgical procedures below the chin should have two preoperative showers with 4% CHG before surgery at a minimum (Mangram *et al.*, 1999).

Multiple studies have demonstrated that the use of CHG preoperatively, post-operatively or with patients at risk has demonstrated either prevention of (or a decrease in) skin to skin microbial contact with bloodborne pathogens. Two showers with 4% CHG were found to result in lower microbial counts than showers with bar soap. Showering or bathing with CHG the night before and morning of surgery provides at least six hours of persistent antimicrobial activity which will be of benefit throughout their surgical procedure (Mangram *et al.*, 1999). The mechanism of washing with a CHG solution and rinsing kills more pathogens than using CHG alone. In a study by Kett *et al.* (2009), the impact of daily skin cleansing of medical intensive care unit patients with a 4% chlorhexidine gluconate (Hibiclens®) was evaluated for the effectiveness in reducing MDROs in MICU patients. The MICU was an 18 bed open bay unit with patients in close proximity. Since 2006, the infection control data collection and reporting has been consistent. Infection control data for the MICU was collected concurrently with clinical care and reviewed retrospectively. Standard precautions (SP) were in place prior to July 2007 and included universal gloving and hand washing before and after patient contact. Tight infection control (TIC) has been advocated since July 2007 and includes SP, improved hand hygiene, full contact precautions, cohorting of patients with multi-drug resistant organisms (MDROs), and twice daily cleaning of all high-touch surfaces. Since July 2008, daily skin cleansing with a 4% CHG (Hibiclens®, Molnlycke Health Care, Norcross, Georgia) in addition to TIC has been instituted. Study results were concluded with a progression of infection control practice from SP to TIC to TIC with CHG was associated with a decrease in MICU patients colonized and/ or infected with multi-drug resistant organisms (MDROs). This data would support additional, multicenter trials evaluating the addition of CHG to tight infection control practices (Kett *et al.*, 2009).

Further evidence suggested by Rao *et al.* (2008) demonstrated that patients undergoing elective total joint arthroplasty (TJA) who used mupirocin ointment to decolonize their nares for *S. Aureus* and who bathed daily with 4% CHG were less prone to postoperative infections. The study used two control groups: 1-no preintervention, and 2-preintervention for *S. aureus* with a decolonization protocol of mupirocin ointment to the nares twice daily, with daily 4% CHG solution bathing for 5 days before surgery. Results indicated all 164 patients in the preintervention group had no postoperative surgical site infections at the end of year one. In addition, the data from the study suggest preoperative decolonization is a safe strategy to reduce *S. aureus* SSIs in patients undergoing TJA and may translate to economic savings to the facility (Rao *et al.*, 2008).

12.3.2.3. Personal Protective Equipment

The use of personal protective equipment (PPE) is considered Standard Precaution in all surgical locations. This includes wearing two pairs of surgical gloves (AORN recommends double gloving on all surgical procedures with a colored underglove that will demonstrate a color indication if the glove is breached), a face mask, sterile gown, and eye wear (goggles or face shields) during surgical procedures. In the non-sterile environment, this includes wearing non-sterile gloves since the potential for contact with blood, body fluids, non-intact skin and contaminated equipment is possible with all patients (AORN, 2011b).

12.3.2.4. Continuing Education

In order to ensure adequate and up to date training, the ASC should employ at least one dedicated person in charge of infection prevention.

12.3.2.5. Documentation

A first and important step for any ASC is to maintain and document appropriately all measures that will identify the ASC as one following Medicare's Condition for Coverage policy.

12.4. INFECTION CONTROL MONITORING

An assessment of nearly 70 ambulatory surgical centers in three states found that lapses in infection control were common, including practices such as hand hygiene, injections, medication safety and equipment reprocessing (Schaeffer *et al.*, 2010). Between June and October 2008, sixty-eight ASC's were assessed; 32 in Maryland, 16 in North Carolina, and 20 in Oklahoma. Five areas of infection control were studied:

• hand hygiene
• injection safety and medication handling
• equipment reprocessing
• environmental cleaning
• handling of blood glucose monitoring equipment

Of the ASC's surveyed, 67.6 % (46/68) had at least 1 lapse in infection control and 17.6% of the facilities had 3 lapses or more of the 5 infection control categories. Subsequently, the facilities involved were required to develop a correctional plan to address deficiencies and submit their plan of action to the State Survey Agency for review. Failure to do so would deem the ASC ineligible for Medicare reimbursement (Schaeffer *et al.*, 2010).

12.5. ACTIVE PARTICIPATION

A comprehensive ASC infection control program includes the environmental, physical and general healthcare provider clinical practices. For proficiency and compliance, the ASC program should include the guidelines recommended by the governing National Expert Committees from the Centers for Disease Control (CDC) on Surgical Site Infections, and the AORN Perioperative Standards and Recommended Practices. In order to maintain an effective and quality ASC program, the following should be initiated:

1. Employ a dedicated Infection Prevention coordinator to:
   • Direct an infection prevention program
   • Deliver appropriate staff training
   • Determine when infection prevention updates are warranted
   • Delegate specific infection control tasks to staff members
2. Develop and employ a monthly infection prevention checklist

- Evaluate the effectiveness of staff hand hygiene practices
- Effectiveness of equipment cleaning
- Review of daily records to ensure that patients completed two 4% CHG baths prior to surgery
- Appropriateness of staff and visitor surgical attire
- Cleanliness of operating room, scrub sink area, storage areas, sterile process and decontamination areas

3. Implement appropriate documentation for standard daily audits
   - Daily air flow exchanges
   - Daily humidity and temperature checks
   - Flash sterilization-how often was it done and was there appropriate documentation
   - Terminal cleaning schedule

All of the above activities should be monitored, evaluated quarterly, corrected and reported as required by accreditation (Evans, 2009).

12.6. LONG-TERM INFECTION CONTROL PRINCIPLES IN AMBULATORY SURGICAL SETTINGS

The number of outpatient ambulatory surgical services continues to increase as new non-invasive surgical technologies expand. Increased use of invasive devices for surgical procedures provides new and challenging risks for infection prevention. Risks associated with contaminated equipment and supplies can be decreased by updated knowledge and the implementation of aseptic techniques and disinfection practices. The challenge to infection prevention and the ambulatory surgery staff is to remain updated and focused on the emerging technologies that may increase the likelihood of preventing HAIs and providing safe patient care. More patients with a high acuity of illness are now being treated in ambulatory surgery centers versus inpatient hospital settings, and often these patients wait for prolonged periods of time and are in close proximity to others. The risk of communicable disease transmission and the presence of multidrug-resistant organisms necessitate that strict infection control standards be maintained in ASCs.

The HCPs, patients, and family members of patients need to be educated to support patient safety and minimize the risk for cross contamination and infection. The Infection Preventionist—or, in some ASCs, the nurse who has been designated with the role of quality control and infection prevention—has unique challenges in continuously providing the ASC infection prevention and regulatory strategies.

With the ever-increasing financial pressure to maintain cost-effective healthcare, freestanding surgical centers continue to be targeted. Today, we have to be diligent in our ability to provide safe, effective and quality care within the ASCs. As more and more ASCs perform surgical procedures once only performed in hospital settings, our ability to keep patients and staff free from blood borne pathogen transmission and postoperative infections becomes an even greater task.

Ann did some additional literature reviews and felt that she could provide appropriate advice. She would instruct her aunt to use 4% CHG soap prior to her surgical procedure. Her aunt was assured that 4% CHG soap can be used the same as other liquid soaps. Ann pointed out the safety-warning label that would discuss avoidance of the certain body parts (especially eyes, ears and genital area) (Table 12.1).

Infection prevention procedures are simple, effective and inexpensive. In the ASC, infectious pathogens can be transmitted through the external environment, instrumentation or inappropriate device cleaning. Additionally, any breach via the mucous membranes, broken skin due to an incision, a needle stick injury or any invasive procedure may provide the route for the transmission of an infection. Following updated guidelines to ensure Standard of Care practices are performed for all procedures for all patients clears the path for Ambulatory Surgery Center care in the future. When patients arrive clean and in good health they have a greater chance for positive surgical outcomes. Taking a bath may sound too simple to discuss; however, general skin cleansing prior to a surgical procedure has the potential to prevent skin infections, thus reducing the risk of cross-infection or a surgical site infection.

12.7. SUMMARY POINTS

- Providing a safe and sanitary environment can prevent the transmission of blood borne pathogens during a surgical procedure in an ASC.
- Adherence to infection control standards consistent with in-patient

hospital guidelines protects the patient, family and healthcare workers.

- Using preventive skin washes (CHG baths) provides added barrier protection against the transmission of blood borne pathogens.
- The maintenance of quality control records provides consistency in reviewing infection control standards associated with surgical equipment, instruments and the quality of airflow.

TABLE 12.1. Guide To General Skin Cleansing At Home.

Good hygiene, such as frequent hand washing and daily skin cleansing, leads to good health. Daily skin cleansing helps to remove microbes and pathogens that may cause diseases.

Pre-operative General Skin Cleansing Instructions for Bathing or Showers

Before you bathe or shower:
- Read the instructions given to you by your healthcare practitioner, and begin your general skin cleansing protocol as directed.
- Carefully read all directions on the product label.
- CHG is not to be used on the face, including around the eyes and ears.
- CHG is not to be applied directly to the genital area.

Night Before Surgery and/or Procedure:
- If you plan to wash your hair, do so with your regular shampoo. Then rinse hair and body thoroughly to remove any shampoo residue.
- Wash your face with your regular soap or water only.
- Thoroughly rinse your body with warm water from the neck down.
- Apply just enough CHG to cover your skin from the neck down to the waist, about
- 1/4 of a 4 oz. bottle. Apply CHG to the skin with a clean washcloth and wash gently.
- Rinse thoroughly with warm water.
- Apply CHG to your skin from the waist down using just enough to cover the unwashed skin, about 1/4 of a 4 oz. bottle, in the same manner as above.
- Rinse thoroughly with warm water
- Do not use your regular soap after applying and rinsing CHG.
- After rinsing, gently pat skin dry with a clean towel.

Morning of Surgery and/or Procedure:
- Shower/bathe again using CHG in the same method as described above using the remaining 1/2 of the 4 oz. bottle.
- Do not apply any lotions, deodorants, powders or perfumes to the body areas that have been cleaned with CHG.

Note: Please include any additional directives as indicated from your healthcare worker. Avoid using CHG around eyes, ears, mucous membranes and genitalia.

Sorrentino, S. (2006). Assisting with Patient Care. St Louis, MO: Mosby, pp. 305–310. American Red Cross. (2009). Modified Bed Bath, Skill 12, Maryland. Followed by the Maryland Board of Nursing. Baltimore City Community College and Harford Community Nursing Assistant training.

12.8. REFERENCES

AORN. (2011a). Perioperative Standards and Recommended Practices; Surgical Attire, pp. 57–71.

AORN. (2011b). Perioperative Standards and Recommended Practices; Skin Antisepsis, pp. 361–379.

Barie, P. (2010). Infection control practices in ambulatory surgical centers. *JAMA,* *303*(22): 2295–2297.

CDC. (2011). Guide to Infection Prevention in Outpatient Settings: Minimum Expectations for Safe Care, pp. 1–15.

CMS (Centers for Medicare and Medicaid Services). 2009. Flash Sterilization Clarification—FY 2010 Ambulatory Surgical Center (ASC) Surveys.

Evans, G. (2009) Effective implementation of Medicare's new infection control program. Focus, March/April 2009, pp. 42–47.

Gerber, C.P. and Kennedy, D. (2007) Enteric virus survival during household laundering and impact of disinfection with sodium hypochlorite. *Appl. Environ. Microbiol.,* *73*(14): 4425–8.

Kett, D.H., Tamayo, M., *et al.* (2009) Impact of Daily Skin Cleansing of Medical Intensive Care Unit Patients with a 4% Chlorhexidine Gluconate (Hibiclens®) on the Incidence of Hospital Acquired Multidrug Resistant Organisms. University of Miami, Poster Presentation. Philadelphia: Infectious Disease Society of America (IDSA).

Manchikanti, L., Parr, A., *et al.* (2011) Ambulatory surgery centers and interventional techniques: a look at long term survival. *Pain Physician, 14*:E177–E215.

Mangram, A.J., Horan, T.C., Pearson, M.L., *et al.* (1999) Guideline for prevention of surgical site infection, 1999. Hospital Infection Control Practices Advisory Committee. *Infect Control Hosp. Epidemiol. 20*(4): 250–78.

NFPA. (2005) 99 Standard for Health Care Facilities. Quincy, MA; National Fire Protection Association.

Phillips, N., Berry, E. and Kohn, M. (2012). Berry & Kohn's Operating Room Technique, pp. 263–266.

Rao, N., Cannella, B., Crosset, L., Yates, A.J. and McGough, R.A. (2008) Preoperative decolonization protocol for Staphlyococcus aureus prevents orthopedic infections. *Clinical Orthopedics and Related Research, 46*(6): 1343–1348.

Schaeffer, M., *et al.* (2010) Infection control assessment of ambulatory centers. *JAMA, 303*(22): 2273–2279.

U.S. Department of Health and Human Services. (2011) Report To Congress. Medicare Ambulatory Surgery Center Value-Based Purchasing Implementation Plan.

CHAPTER 13

Infection Control in the Community

JEANETTE ADAMS PhD., RN

This chapter will focus on the basic infection control practices that advance practice healthcare professionals need to know about the transmission of communicable infections such as Methicillin Resistant Staphylococcus Aureus (MRSA), Clostridium difficile (c.diff) and Human immunodeficiency virus/Acquired immunodeficiency syndrome (HIV/AIDS). A simple case of community-acquired infections will be presented to emphasize the important issues associated with safety and further transmission of community-acquired infections.

13.1. CASE PRESENTATION

Folorunso is a 36-year-old Nigerian national who came to the United States of America (USA) to attend a University. He was granted an education visa. He has been in the USA for two years. During the summer he traveled to Nigeria to visit his family and homeland. He applied and was granted a visa for his family to live in the USA. He and his wife, Katherine, have three children, ages 15, 11, and 7 years old. They reside in a family dormitory on the University campus. The living quarters have two bedrooms, one bathroom, a galley kitchen and a small living room. His children will be going to public school—one in high school, one in middle school and one in elementary school. His wife has found employment at a local cafeteria. She works in the kitchen with food preparation, cooking and serving. At the end of the day from work, Katherine is allowed to take the leftover food home to her family. The family does not own a car and relies on public transportation. The children use the school bus for transportation to their schools. Katherine takes the public bus to the restaurant and for grocery shopping.

When Katherine enrolled her children in public school, she was required to submit a vaccination and immunization record. The children had not received the required vaccinations that the school required. Katherine did not want her children to receive the vaccines for fear of them getting an infectious disease. She does not believe the children should receive the vaccine.

Folorunso was diagnosed with human immunodeficiency virus (HIV) five years ago. He is monitored by a healthcare professional with an antiviral regimen. Since Katherine has moved to the USA, she has been feeling tired and is susceptible to colds and flus. She has made an appointment with a health care clinic for evaluation.

13.2. ESSENTIAL CONTENT FOR INFECTION CONTROL SKILLS

Community health can be related to local, regional, national and even global populations. Health care outside controlled settings pose a challenge to health care professionals. The health care professional must possess skills to recognize vulnerabilities that predispose the community to infections. There are regulations in place with governmental agencies that promote safeguards to inhibit, prevent and contain transmission of infectious agents. The health care professional must possess competencies in the area of detection, surveillance and education in infection prevention and control within the community. This chapter provides information for the health care professional to consider when providing infection control strategies for the community.

His wife has found employment at a local cafeteria. She works in the kitchen with food preparation, cooking and serving. At the end of the day from work, Katherine is allowed to take the leftover food home to her family . . . Katherine takes the public bus to the restaurant and for grocery shopping.

13.3. FOOD BORNE INFECTIONS

The United States Department of Agriculture (USDA) plays a major role in promoting food safety for the community. The Food Safety and Inspection Service (FSIS) is responsible for the safety of meat, poultry and egg products (FSIS, 2012). Processing, temperature and delivery of our food products are regulated to prevent and minimize the transmission of bacteria, toxins, parasites, viruses and protozoa. *Salmonella*, a gram negative bacteria, accounts for more than 50% of food borne illnesses and *Campylobacter*, also a gram negative bacteria, is the 2nd most common bacteria responsible for foodborne illnesses. *Escherichia coli, listeria monocytogenes, staphylococcus aureus, clostridium perfringens* and *clostridium botulinum* comprise the other common organisms prone to cause infectious illnesses from food sources (FSIS, 2012).

Strategies to minimize the introduction and proliferation of infectious agents aim at the entire food safety chain, including farmers, industry, and food inspecting retailers, food service workers and consumers. Health care professionals' role is with education of communities in food safety. The FSIS provides the Clean, Separate, Cook and Chill framework for food safety education (FSIS, 2012).

Cleanliness is of primary importance when working with food products. Hands must be washed before and after handling raw foods and before consuming food. The preparation area must be cleaned with hot, soapy water or disinfectant with paper towels that are immediately discarded after use. If reusable cloth towels or rags are used, they should be washed in hot water, detergent and bleach. Once cloths or towels are used to clean the preparation of one food source, they are considered contaminated and either discarded or placed for laundry. A new cloth/towel should be used for each food product during preparation.

Separation of food products is necessary to avoid cross-contamination. Food products such as meat, fish and poultry may leak fluid to other food sources or transfer bacteria if placed on same surface. A cutting board should be cleaned with hot, soapy water between each food product to avoid cross contamination. Cooking raw food is necessary to promote food safety. A food thermometer should be used to ensure meat and poultry are at the recommended temperatures (Food Safety, 2012). Raw milk and unpasteurized dairy products should be avoided.

Food safety also includes strategies for cooked food. Chilling cooked food within two hours at room temperature minimizes the proliferation of bacterial growth. In addition, frozen food should be thawed within refrigeration and not at room temperature. Leftover foods should be properly heated and sauces should be brought to a boil prior to eating. Leftovers left in refrigeration should be discarded after two days, as these food products may be unsafe. Whenever in doubt, it is best to err on the side of safety.

When Katherine enrolled her children in public school, she was required to submit a vaccination and immunization record. The children had not received the required vaccinations that the school required. Katherine did not want her children to receive the vaccines for fear of them getting an infectious disease. She does not believe the children should receive the vaccine.

13.4. PREVENTION OF INFECTIOUS DISEASES

13.4.1. Immunizations

Immunity is a strategy used to protect and prevent infectious diseases. Immunization is the process of creating antibodies to fight infectious diseases. Vaccines are an artificial passive immunization. Many infectious diseases are controlled with the institution of vaccines (NIAID, 2012). Vaccines contain a weakened or killed infectious agent. When the vaccine is given to the individual, the immune system responds by developing an antibody to attack and rid the body of the infectious agent. These antibodies have the ability to recognize the infectious agent whenever the body has exposure and triggers the antibodies to attack again. As a result, immunity is established for this infectious agent.

Community immunity plays an important role in containing infectious agents within a population. If most of the members of the community receive immunizations against contagious infections, there are fewer outbreaks within the community. Fewer outbreaks decrease the likelihood of exposure for those who are not immunized within the community. This provides protection of vulnerable populations within the community who are not candidates for immunization because of their compromised immune system (NIAID, 2012).

Immunizations and vaccines are an essential strategy to contain, control and prevent contagious infectious diseases. The Centers for Disease Control and Prevention (CDC) provide recommendations for vaccines from infants to children. Health care professionals need protection from additional infectious agents since they are prone to more frequent exposure and potential for transmission (CDC, 2012). For people who travel outside the USA, the CDC has recommendations for immunizations and vaccines to specific countries. There are required immunizations and vaccines for entry into the USA. The CDC provides travel information to promote health and protection with travel notices of infectious diseases and problems putting travelers at risk. Health care professionals are responsible for being compliant to vaccines for the welfare of themselves as well as the public. Health care professionals must be knowledgeable of vaccines and immunizations so that they can convey the significance in infectious disease control and prevention.

He and his wife, Katherine, have three children, ages 15, 11, and 7 years old. They reside in a family dormitory on the University campus. The living quarters have two bedrooms, one bathroom, a galley kitchen and a small living room.

13.4.2. Shared Living Conditions

Infection prevention and control in communities involve residential environments. Residential environments vary from spacious dwellings to crowded living spaces. People living in a confined space have a greater risk of transmitting contagious infections. *Mycobacterium tuberculosis* is an airborne infectious disease that is transmitted through coughing and sputum. A primary intervention is to protect other people from contracting the infection through initiation of pharmacological therapy to combat the bacteria. Members within the residence should stay away until the active phase of tuberculosis (TB) is contained. Other strategies of protection include cough and sputum hygiene, wearing a mask when around others, ventilation of the room and most important, completing the medications regime prescribed (CDC, 2012).

Bacterial meningitis is another highly contagious infection for shared living environments. Those most at risk for meningococcal meningitis are persons living in college dormitories and the military. Bacterial meningitis is transmitted through close contact with oral secretions such as kissing. Early recognition and treatment with antibiotics are essential (CDC, 2012).

13.4.3. Public Facilities

Public facilities are an inherent source of pathogens for communities and contribute to transmission of infectious agents. Schools, restaurants, transportation, recreation and entertainment are shared public facilities that most people use on a regular basis. Schools are a vibrant place for the transmission of viruses such as colds and flu. Restaurants rely on employee adherence to infection control and hand hygiene to prevent transmission of Hepatitis and viruses. Public transportation such as buses, trains or airplanes creates an environment of crowded, contained spaces that promote transmission of infections. Recreation playgrounds and sports facilities allow many people to handle shared equipment as well as doorknobs, handrails and restrooms. Public showers contribute to fungal transmissions such as "athlete's foot." Camps and schools are common facilities where ringworm, another fungal infection, is commonly seen. Ringworm, known as tinea, is very contagious and may be contracted from beauty salons, pets and those who share personal items such as hairbrushes and combs, personal clothing or bed linens (CDC, 2012). Venues that contain animal exhibits or petting zoos are potential activities that may promote the transmission of *E. coli* from animals to humans, especially small children who may unconsciously place their hands in their mouths after touching the animal or their surroundings. Good hand hygiene should be employed to prevent these transmissions (CDC, 2012).

13.5. METHICILLIN RESISTANT STAPHYLOCOCCUS AUREUS (MRSA)

Staphylococcus Aureus is a common bacterium found on skin and mucous membranes. MRSA is a *staphylococcus aureus* strain that is not responsive to antibiotics. MRSA was most often limited to healthcare settings until the mid-1990s, when MRSA was identified in the community in healthy persons without any contact with healthcare settings (CDC, 2012). When community MRSA (CA-MRSA, as it is known) started, distinct characteristics of the bacteria were displayed that were not found in MRSA acquired from healthcare associated infections (HAI-MRSA). However, these characteristics are becoming less distinct as more CA-MRSA increases (CDC, 2012). Transmission of CA-MRSA is commonly seen in athletes, schools, prisons, military personnel and persons living in crowded, close living quarters. Although HAI-MRSA is showing a downward trend, CA-MRSA is showing an upward growth (CDC, 2012). Most CA-MRSA involves skin infections and is readily resolved.

Hand hygiene is a primary strategy for prevention and containment. Any draining wounds should be cleaned and dressed using protective precautions and medical asepsis. Contaminated dressings should be discarded in a closed container to prevent contact with others. Healthcare professionals need to continue surveillance and monitoring as well as encourage affected persons to seek healthcare treatment.

13.6. *CLOSTRIDIUM DIFFICILE* (*C-diff.*)

Clostridium difficile (C-diff.) is a well-documented health care associated infection developed as a result of antimicrobial therapy, which reduces the normal flora in the bowel and allows overgrowth of *C-diff.* (CDC, 2012). Community associated clostridium difficile-associated diarrhea (CA-CDAD) started being reported in the mid-2000s. Individuals were developing CA-CDAD who were otherwise healthy, without diagnosis of disease or illness. CA-CDAD is not associated with antimicrobial therapy. Unlike typical patient population for healthcare-related *C-diff.* such as the elderly, trends among individuals with CA-CDAD are young adults with no history of antimicrobial use (Khana, *et al.*, 2012). There is controversy as to what causes CA-CDAD. Recent studies have conflicting results with limitations of operational definitions for CA-CDAD. More studies are needed to clarify the epidemiology of CA-CDAD (Gouliouris, Forsyth, and Brown, 2009). Surveillance and monitoring of CA-CDAD shows growth in the past few years among certain community groups (Freeman *et al.*, 2010).

Folorunso was diagnosed with HIV five years ago. He is followed by a healthcare professional with an antiviral regimen. Since Katherine has moved to the USA, she has been feeling tired and is susceptible to colds and flus. She has made an appointment with a health care clinic for evaluation.

13.7. HUMAN IMMUNODEFICIENCY VIRUS (HIV)

Human immunodeficiency virus is a retrovirus that can be transmitted through blood and body secretions (CDC, 2012). The virus attacks the immune system with a target on CD4 T cells, macrophages and dendritic cells.

In the community environment, the focus is on prevention of transmission with education on safe sexual practices, maintaining medication regime, single needle usage and protective personal equipment. There is an increase in the number of people who have HIV and are living with AIDS. In fact, most individuals who are diagnosed with HIV are considered to have a chronic disease that is treatable with antiviral medications. The morbidity and mortality of people living with HIV has drastically changed since the diagnosis of disease. Therefore, most individuals living with HIV have assimilated within their communities and lead productive lives. The most important principle for individuals about HIV/AIDS is to use prevention methods so that the virus is not transmitted to others.

13.8. INTERPRETATION/APPLICATION OF INFECTION CONTROL DATA

Food borne illnesses can be difficult to diagnose. Typically, these illnesses appear as flu-like symptoms and diarrhea. They are more severe in vulnerable populations related to age, immunosuppressed or immunocompromised and who have existing illnesses. There are several agencies in the USA that focus on safety for the American population. These include the public health system, CDC, USDA, American Blood Bank and the World Health Organization. Immunizations and vaccines control transmission of several infectious diseases in the USA. Vaccines prevent diseases that can be deadly or cause permanent disabilities to the body. Transmission of infections is facilitated by human contact and close proximity. Hand hygiene is the first line of prevention of transmission. Knowledge of the epidemiology of the infectious agent and the mode of transmission enables the healthcare professional to provide essential education in containing the spread of the infection.

13.9. DISCUSSION ABOUT PATIENT SAFETY AND HEALTH SYSTEM ISSUES RELATED TO ICP

Community settings are unique in the fact that we must all be diligent in practicing infection prevention. Each individual carries a burden of responsibility to keep the environment conducive to healthy living. It only takes one outbreak to place the community at risk. The CDC provides guidelines and recommendations for infection control and prevention. Education is a vital component for the health care professional.

Specific strategies that may be used to provide healthy communities include as affordable, safe, and accessible housing, and the ability to enhance the infrastructure for public or community health centers that provide data to prevent communicable diseases. Other important issues include the integration of technology that provides data analysis related to the health of the population, the ability to cross-train health care staff and the use of shared databases that can predict the needs of a community population.

13.10. SUMMARY POINTS

- Community settings are relatively uncontrolled environments that facilitate transmission of infections.
- Hygiene is essential to prevent transmission of infections.
- The individual in the community is a vital component in the cycle of infection prevention.
- Vaccine compliance promotes the control and prevention of infectious disease for the community.
- The closer proximity of people increases the likelihood of infection transmission.
- Community associated infections are becoming more prevalent in the absence of healthcare related settings.

13.11. REFERENCES

Centers for Disease Control & Prevention, "Vaccine schedules," accessed, 8/12/12: http://www.cdc.gov/vaccines/schedules/

Centers for Disease Control & Prevention, "Bacterial Meningitis," accessed 8/12/12: http://www.cdc.gov/meningitis/bacterial.html

Centers for Disease Control & Prevention, "Dermatophytes," accessed 8/12/12: http://www.cdc.gov/fungal/dermatophytes/

Centers for Disease Control & Prevention, "Healthy pets, healthy people," accessed 8/12/12: http://www.cdc.gov/healthypets/diseases/ecoli.htm

Centers for Disease Control & Prevention, "Community associated MRSA," accessed 8/12/12: http://epi.publichealth.nc.gov/cd/diseases/mrsa_ca.html

Centers for Disease Control & Prevention, "Tuberculosis," accessed 8/12/12: http://www.cdc.gov/tb/

Freeman, J., Bauer, M. P., Baines, S. D., Cover, J., Fawley, W. N., Goorhuis, B., Kuiper, E. J., & Wilcox, M. H. (2010). The changing epidemiology of clostridium difficile infections. *Clin. Microbiol. Rev., 23*(3): 529–549.

Food Safety and Inspection Service, National Advisory Committee on Meat and Poultry Inspection. [Docket No. FSIS-2012-0030]; Federal Register Volume 77, Number 152; accessed 8/12/12: http://www.FSIS.usada.gov

Food Safety: "Cooking at the right temperature." Aaccessed 8/12/12: http://www.foodsafety.gov/keep/basics/cook/index.html

Gouliouris, T., Forsyth, D. R., & Brown, N. M. (2009). Clostridium difficile-associated diarrhoea (CDAD): new and contentious issues. *Age & Ageing 38*(5): 497–500.

Khana, S., Pardi, D. S., Aronson, S. L., Kramer, P. P., Orenstein, R., St. Sauver, J. L., Harmsen, W. S., Zinsmeister, A. R. (2012) The epidemiology of community acquired clostridium difficile infection: a population based study. *American Journal of Gastroenterology,* January *107*(1): 89–95.

National Institutes of Allergy & Infectious Diseases, "Herd Immunity," accessed 8/12/12: http://www.niaid.nih.gov/topics/pages/communityimmunity.aspx

CHAPTER 14

Infection Control for Emergency Mobile Health Units

MICHELLE WRIGHT MS., RN, DOCTORAL STUDENT

The intent of this chapter will be to address the major infection control issues associated with emergency mobile health units needed for rapid deployment to natural and man-made catastrophes. The chapter will use a public health case study exemplifying needed infection control practices focusing on transmission, and include issues related to resources, protection and contamination.

14.1. CASE PRESENTATION

Joan Smith is a nurse practitioner who works with an orthopedic surgery team that specializes in spinal surgeries. While Joan is getting ready for work, she hears on the news that a massive earthquake has occurred in the Indian Ocean and a tsunami has caused devastation in Sri Lanka, India, and Thailand. Joan has gone on relief efforts after hurricane Katrina and the earthquake in Haiti as a nurse, and recalls previous devastation to the same area in 2004. She is keenly aware that trauma is one of the main causes of morbidity and mortality when disasters caused by tsunamis occur and specialty services offered by her team will be needed. When she arrives to work, she is not surprised to find out her team has been approached to assist relief efforts and is happy to help those desperately in need. Joan is concerned for how she can help keep herself healthy, as she inadvertently contracted Cholera when she was working in Haiti after the earthquake. She assumes conditions may be similar and she is unaware what communicable diseases are endemic in Thailand where her team will be providing services.

Prior to leaving the States, Joan has an appointment with the travel medicine specialist at her hospital to obtain information

215

about endemic diseases and vaccinations she should receive before traveling. The visit is required by the hospital to decrease risks to provider health while offering aid, but Joan is warned immunity may not be acquired for a number of weeks. Because of this, the doctor reminds Joan to wash her hands frequently and to teach patients, family, and staff around her to do the same, since hand hygiene is still the best method of preventing infection, even in disasters. Since Joan's team will be working in Thailand, malaria prophylaxis is recommended. Joan states she will use repellant that is made with DEET, wear long sleeves and pants, and sleep under nets to prevent being bitten by mosquitoes.

When Joan arrives in Thailand, she is relieved to see the temporary hospital was built on the side of a hill where it cannot be reached by residual floodwater. Joan notices there are some latrines located near the entrance of the facility and is alarmed when she notices there are no hand hygiene stations or hand sanitizer available near the facilities. Joan immediately asks the nurse triaging patients if anything is available for people to wash their hands near the latrines. The nurse tells Joan to ask the director of the unit because they are in control of resources and their distribution since everything is so scarce. Joan finds the director and explains her concern for the unsanitary conditions, particularly because of her previous experience with the Cholera epidemic in Haiti. The director is thankful for Joan's observation and states hand sanitizer stations will be set up immediately, as they were supposed to be set up already and must have gotten lost in the chaos.

As Joan is assessing and treating patients, she notices that family members routinely provide basic care for their relatives and nearby patients. She also notices there is extreme crowding and hardly any water available. Joan knows both situations create the potential to accelerate the spread of infection. She works with other staff and volunteers to create signs illustrating when hand hygiene is needed and teaches all patients and family members at every encounter to wash their hands after using the restroom, as well as before and after eating or touching others.

The team Joan is working with also receives patients from a different disaster facility that only performs surgeries and immediate postoperative care, so that surgery can be performed on as many injured people as possible. Her newest patient arrives, and in addition to crush injuries to bilateral lower extremities, he has a persistent dry cough, diminished breath sounds, and fever.

The patient denies having asthma or respiratory issues. He stated he has had a cough for a few months and sometimes wakes up in a cold sweat. Joan consults with the medical personnel from the sending facility and they deny traumatic intubation of the patient for the surgical procedure. They stated that the patient had a cough upon arrival, but they had not taken a chest radio-graph because it was unavailable and his laboratory values were consistent with what you would expect in trauma patients. Joan decided to administer a Tuberculin Skin Test, place a surgical mask on herself and the patient since there were no N95 masks, and moved the patient to one of the two respiratory isolation rooms because she knows that tuberculosis has been endemic in Thailand.

14.2. ESSENTIAL CONTENT FOR INFECTION CONTROL SKILLS

Increased mobility in society creates new challenges to preventing infections more than ever before. Natural and manmade disasters re-quiring healthcare workers from around the world to come together and render aid to those in need have been occurring in recent years with alarming frequency. Current literature offers insight into infection con-trol issues encountered in areas affected by war and other catastrophic events. When care is provided in areas outside a practitioner's regular domain, additional barriers will be encountered. Particularly poignant issues are unsanitary conditions, lack of supplies, overcrowding, and the need to diagnose disease without laboratory data. This chapter will address these issues and provide practitioners with strategies for pre-venting the spread of infection during a natural or man-made disaster.

14.2.1. Site Selection

When Joan arrives in Thailand, she is relieved to see the tem-porary hospital they built is situated on the side of a hill where it cannot be reached by residual floodwater. Joan notices there are some latrines located near the entrance of the facility . . .

When selecting a site for an emergency mobile health unit, terrain and regular weather patterns for the area should be considered. Ide-ally, the site will be on higher ground to avoid flooding in the event of inclement weather. If an area on a plateau is available, it would be ideal since it would allow for easy drainage and easier to create paths for unsanitary waste to drain away from treatment areas. Swampy areas should be avoided. When a site is placed near a river, additional emphasis should be placed on utilizing available restrooms—and not the waterway—in order to prevent polluting water that may be used downstream by other members of the population. If there is an area with nearby trees, they may be helpful in shielding the site from wind and sun, and in reducing dust. Local authorities in the area should be consulted because situating a facility too close to a wooded area may be dangerous due to local fauna and possible enemies if it is a war-torn area. Additionally, the site should be easily accessible so that supplies can be delivered for the utilization of local services. When constructing the unit, the entryways should not face downwind since it may increase risk of vector borne illnesses (Connolly, 2005).

14.2.2. Unsanitary Conditions

When Joan arrives in Thailand, she is alarmed when she notices there are no hand hygiene stations or hand sanitizer available near the latrines . . . and explains her concern for the unsanitary conditions, particularly because of her previous experience with the Cholera epidemic in Haiti.

Many times, communities in dire need may not have had good sanitation infrastructure prior to a disaster. For example, before the 2010 earthquake in Haiti, a majority of the population did not have sufficient sanitation facilities and less than half had clean water prior to the earthquake (Lichtenberger et al., 2010). Lack of reliable pre-existing systems may require workers to create a way to keep sewage from safe water, food, and human contact. Additionally, as in the case of hurricane Katrina, existing infrastructure may be completely decimated and alternatives must be used.

14.2.3. Lack of Toilets

Indiscriminant defecation must be prohibited. Signs and fences should be placed to protect areas uphill from treatment areas or near food and water supplies to prevent contamination. The use of portable latrines is likely in disaster situations. The World Health Organization recommends an initial goal of 1 latrine for 50 people and to provide additional latrines when available. Ideally, there will be at least 1 latrine for every 20 people (Connolly, 2005). Careful attention should be paid to where the toilets are placed in relation to patient care areas. Facilities for patients and families should be located near entrances for easy usage. This also allows for use of latrines by patients, families, and others awaiting care or admission. Separate facilities can be established at an alternate location for staff. It is advisable to have separate facilities for healthcare providers and patients with diarrhea, since it may be infectious in nature. Staff and patients that develop diarrhea while in the mobile health unit should be monitored closely (Lichtenberger *et al.*, 2010).

14.2.4. Lack of Hand Hygiene Facilities

Since disasters frequently disturb existing water supplies, alternative methods of hand sanitation must be used. Alcohol-based hand sanitizers have been used successfully by placing dispensers throughout tents and by educating patients, family members and healthcare providers how and when they should be used. Particular attention should be paid to visitors and family members (since they frequently help provide care for family members) and patients close in proximity to their family member when in disaster situations (Lichtenberger *et al.*, 2010). Great care should be taken to educate people to use the sanitizer before and after patient contact, before mealtimes, and after using bathroom facilities. It may be useful to create signs that include pictures encouraging hand hygiene, especially if it is not a normal practice for the culture in the affected area.

14.2.5. Personal Hygiene Measures

When disasters strike, personal hygiene frequently falls down on the list of priorities even though it is paramount for preventing soft tissue infection and preventing outbreaks of vectors such as lice and scabies. When personal bathing facilities are established, they will probably use chlorinated nonpotable water and may be of limited supply. Attention should be paid to the direction of drainage flow from the shower facility to ensure a reservoir is not being created and that waste products are flowing away from patients and staff to prevent cross-contamination.

Hygiene issues associated with immobile patients must be considered. Often times in disaster situations, hygiene will be performed by family members or untrained volunteers who must be taught where to obtain proper water and where to dispose of waste water. Water should not be haphazardly thrown into open areas or where it may collect into pools, since it can be a breeding ground for bacteria and infectious vectors like mosquitoes. Family should be taught that any items contaminated with blood should be disposed of in marked biohazard containers to be incinerated.

14.2.6. Sterilization Issues

When disasters occur and mobile units are created, there will be limited equipment and electricity. Autoclaves or other gas sterilization machines will not be available, so instruments and other equipment used for multiple patients will need to be cleaned in bleach or alcohol baths. Sterilization of instruments has been effective in recent disasters (Lichtenberger et al., 2010). After the January 2010 earthquake in Haiti, Wang (2010) reported only 2 out of 15 patients had developed infection or wound breakdown by May 2010 after instruments were sterilized with bleach and alcohol. Follow-up data on patient outcomes in disaster situation is limited because patients rarely return for follow-up care or receive care from other providers after the initial stabilization period.

14.2.7. Disposing of Biohazards

Materials that contain blood or other infectious bodily fluids should be disposed of and incinerated when possible. The waste should not be stored in a location near the hospital or where food is prepared to help prevent contamination of the food supply. The location should be secure so that members of the population will not be able to search through trash and inadvertently be exposed to infectious waste (Lichtenberger et al., 2010). Non-medical waste should also be treated with care to avoid scavengers. Plastic or metal bins should be used for disposal of all waste products until they can be incinerated or removed.

Bodies and body parts should also be removed from patient care areas and held at an alternate location until they can be transferred to a cemetery or other designated destination. Bodies of patients that die as the result of trauma from the disaster generally have low risk of causing disease outbreaks (Noji, 2005). The corpses should be treated the same as in any other healthcare setting and should be properly identified and stored in another location so that proper funeral arrangements can be made after the situation improves. Patients that succumb to highly infectious diseases should be removed and disposed of as quickly as possible. Patients who die of cholera should be bathed with 2% chlorine solution, orifices should be blocked with cotton wool soaked in the same solution and placed in plastic bags. Patients who perish from typhus should be treated with insecticide and bagged immediately. In the case of viral hemorrhagic fevers, full biohazard practices should be followed. Bodies should be cremated or bagged and buried at least 2 meters below ground. If biohazard body bags are not available, bodies can be wrapped in cloth soaked in formaldehyde and then placed in a plastic bag. All belongings and items that came in contact with the body should be burned (Connolly, 2005). When possible, it is best to incorporate cultural burial rituals; however, when there are high mortality rates it may not be possible. Careful records should be maintained of individuals who succumbed to illness, so that ceremonies may be held after the epidemic but should not be removed from the burial location in the case of highly infectious diseases.

14.2.8. Lack of Aeration

When designing the layout of a mobile health unit, airflow should be considered. It is likely fans and air conditioning will not be available initially. If ventilation is installed in mobile units, direction of airflow should be considered. When there is risk of airborne or droplet transmission of disease and a fixed number of airflow exchanges is not feasible, vents pointed from the ceiling over healthcare providers in the direction of the patient may assist in reducing transmission of diseases to staff. N95 masks for prevention of airborne diseases, like tuberculosis, should be available for use in countries where the disease is prevalent because crowding increases the likelihood the disease will be spread. Surgical masks should also be supplied to patients with symptoms of respiratory illness. When there is threat of airborne illness, active surveillance may be useful in preventing spread of infections. Screening questionnaires can be used when patients arrive, prior to entry into the facility to ensure placement into proper location (Cruz *et al.*, 2010).

14.3. VECTOR BORNE ILLNESSES

Joan decides to administer a Tuberculin Skin Test, places a surgical mask on herself and the patient since there are no N95 masks, and moves the patient to one of the two respiratory isolation rooms because she knows that tuberculosis is endemic in Thailand.

Mosquitoes and flies should be controlled by applying insect repellant with DEET, utilizing mosquito nets impregnated with permethrine and fly traps, eliminating open water reservoirs, spraying for mosquitoes when possible and placing warfarin-based bait to control rodents. Daily fumigation of facilities is advisable whenever possible (Connolly, 2005; Lichtenberger *et al.*, 2010). Body lice can be vectors for typhus, relapsing fever and trench fever. Incoming patients should be inspected for infestations. Infected patients' clothing should be removed and the patients treated with designated insecticides. Good general sanitation will also help control flies capable of spreading diarrheal disease and trachoma. Regular removal of garbage and safe storage of food will help control and prevent any issues with rodents.

14.3.1. Lack of Water

Lack of water for drinking, waste disposal, and hygiene purposes is associated with development of diarrheal illness, skin infections, vector borne disease, and poisoning. If access to water is delayed, an epidemic will almost certainly ensue. The minimal amount of water required is 7 liters (L) per person per day. This only applies during emergency situations and allows for minimal hygiene. Fifty L/person/day is the recommended minimum in general hospital facilities and 100 L/person/day is ideal in surgical and obstetric settings to prevent waterborne communicable diseases. Bottled water should be provided for drinking; if not available, it is important to drink only biologically safe water. Initially, it may be necessary to ration the water supply to ensure all patients have enough for survival. Vegetables that cannot be cleaned properly should not be eaten. As mentioned previously, lack of running water can become a major hygiene issue (Connolly, 2005). It is advisable to have alcohol-based had sanitizer at all toilet facilities, and at entrances to patient care areas and dining locations.

14.3.2. Lack of Food

Food shortage and malnutrition in emergency situations increase acquisition of communicable diseases, particularly in vulnerable populations (Connolly, 2005). In emergency situations, deficiencies in protein, thiamine, niacin, and vitamin C are common. Children are particularly vulnerable to these deficiencies, increasing their risk of acquiring infections with a more severe and prolonged course of illness. Loss of appetite, fever, vomiting, and diarrhea commonly occur with communicable diseases and further exacerbate malnutrition. Care should be taken to assure adequate general rations are provided to patients being cared for based on height and weight. The following general food safety measures should be applied:

- prepare and wash foods using chlorinated water
- ensuring food is covered and stored properly before cooking
- eat prepared foods immediately
- perform proper hand hygiene prior to preparing food and eating
- disinfect food areas daily

14.3.3. Lack of Electrical Power

In many disaster situations, there will likely not be electricity and facilities will be run solely on generators. This limits access to energy available for general and medical purposes. Refrigeration capabilities will be limited, hindering the ability to store food, medications, and laboratory specimens. Alternatives that are stable at ambient temperatures must be considered and used. Lighting for procedures and other medical equipment, such as ventilators, will be limited and may affect patient care and outcomes. Heating and cooling capabilities will also likely be limited, which may contribute to poor patient outcomes by placing additional stress on the patients. Limited power will also limit communication to outside resources via phones, radio, and Internet, increasing the difficulty of coordinating care for persons affected by the disaster (Vane, Winthrop and Martinez, 2010).

14.3.4. Lack of Personal Protective Equipment

Gowns, gloves, masks, and other personal protective equipment (PPE) may be unavailable or limited in quantity. It is important to stress the need for excellent hand hygiene practices and judicious use of available PPE. Resources should not be wasted or reused, particularly if there is a disease outbreak.

14.3.5. Poor Immunization Compliance

In developing countries, immunizations for tetanus may be limited or non-existent, and in developed countries there has been trend in some communities to refuse vaccinations. In disasters where multiple crush injuries, fractures, and contaminated wounds are encountered, the risk of tetanus should always be considered. Immunization and immunoglobulin should be provided based on patient history and wounds should be decontaminated as soon as possible (Waring and Brown, 2005).

14.4. OVERCROWDING

The team Joan is working with also receives patients from a different disaster facility that only performs surgeries and immediate postoperative care, so that surgery can be performed on as many injured people as possible.

14.4.1. Lack of Beds

Field hospitals try to establish 3 feet between patients to reduce the odds of transferring infections, but it is nearly impossible to maintain in disaster situations (Lichtenberger et al., 2010). This issue of concern that contributes the most to overcrowding is the mobile unit's surge capacity (Kris et al., 2010; Rebmann, English and Carrico, 2007). Surge capacity is the ability of a facility to expand care related to demand. Field hospitals and mobile units usually have the minimum staff and resources necessary to provide care. The limited amount of space for treating patients results in difficulty accommodating surge capacity in disasters. When facilities open after a community has been decimated by a disaster, the need for care often outweighs the available resources. Patients must be strictly triaged which can result in ethical and moral dilemmas for providers not normally encountered in their regular practice environment. Patients may need to be discharged earlier in the recovery process in order to free up space for lifesaving procedures, leaving them more prone to complications. Transfer to other facilities—either at the disaster location or facilities outside the disaster zone—may be possible for some patients (Kris et al., 2010). When patients are transferred to other facilities, the accepting facility should be notified of any outbreaks occurring at the sending facility, as well as any suspected infectious disease the patient may have. Additionally, it is best to allow only one family member at the bedside at a time. This will help reduce crowding in already cramped quarters. Requiring both patients and family to wear identification can help staff monitor and regulate crowding (Lichtenberger et al., 2010)

14.4.2. Patient Placement

When setting up a mobile unit or triaging patients, it is important to group patients with care. Units for medical, surgical and pediatric populations should be created when possible, since their needs and predisposition to infections will differ based on clinical presentation. Potentially infectious patients should be isolated with appropriate precautions whenever possible. When this is not possible to isolate patients, patients with similar presentations should be cohorted. In disaster situations, it can be helpful to use color-coded wristbands to assign patients to designated areas. Utilizing such a system makes it clear to everyone coming in contact with the patient where care is to be provided. It should be stressed to the patient and family members to stay in the designated area for their own safety, as well other patients requiring care (Cruz *et al.*, 2010).

14.4.3. Storage Issues

Initially, it may be impossible to refrigerate items or there may be very limited availability of space. As far as food rations, only nonperishable items should be used. Additionally, it is likely that food, water, and medical supplies will all be stored in the same area. Designating certain containers or shelved areas for food or medication may help prevent cross-contamination of items. If possible, it is best to store food and medications in separate locations. It is beneficial to make sure that items are stored on crates or pallets to keep them off the ground where they could easily become contaminated with dirt or ground water that may contain infectious agents (Lichtenberger *et al.*, 2010).

14.5. PERSONNEL SAFETY

Joan is concerned for how she can help keep herself healthy, as she inadvertently contracted Cholera when she was working in Haiti after the earthquake. She assumes conditions may be similar and she is unaware what communicable diseases are endemic in Thailand where her team will be providing services.

Before working in a mobile health unit, precautions should be taken to ensure all worker vaccinations are up to date and that they are in good health. Vaccinations for tetanus, measles, meningitis, yellow fever, and cholera may be needed. Infections caused by these agents are the most common in emergency situations where there is trauma and overcrowding (Connolly, 2005). It is likely that patients will also require the same vaccinations and they should be made available as soon as cold boxes and refrigerators are available for vaccine storage. Mobile health units are physically and emotionally stressful and workers should receive pre-deployment counseling, if possible, prior to travel so they are somewhat prepared for what they will encounter. Post-exposure prophylaxis for hepatitis, HIV and other diseases should be available at the mobile health unit in case workers are exposed while proving care. Personal protective equipment and disposal containers for sharps should be provided. Additionally, staff should be assigned to work in shifts to avoid fatigue and associated medical errors (Lichtenberger *et al.*, 2010).

14.6. MEDICALLY TRAINED VOLUNTEERS

Medically trained personnel typically come from all backgrounds, from emergency to intensive care to orthopedics. Practitioners generally have some understanding of infection control measures; however, they should be briefed on particular challenges they will be faced with when entering a disaster situation and mobile health units. The staff will probably be unfamiliar with diseases endemic to the area if it is not an area in which they normally provide care. Checklists and other quick reference sources will prove useful in preventing errors and improving care for patients in disaster scenarios (Rebmann *et al.*, 2007). Checklists in disaster situations provide a resource for ensuring protocols are followed in a stressful and unfamiliar environment by increasing communication of the team who may not normally work together (Chu, Trelles and Ford, 2011). Checklists were implemented by United States Army nurses in Bosnia in 1996 to ensure essential components of infection control principals, such as surveillance and reporting, were being followed and are still used today (Vane *et al.*, 2010).

Workers should be trained in surveillance techniques so they can identify when epidemics start and be able to contain them. Staff should be educated to report the following illnesses to the medical officer in charge because they are frequently associated with epidemics in disasters:

- diarrhea
- suspected lower respiratory infections
- measles

- meningitis
- infectious diseases endemic to the disaster area like malaria or Lassa fever

Appropriate isolation measures should be initiated if necessary and feasible. Frequently in disaster situations, laboratory confirmation is not available or will not be timely. When this situation occurs, patients should be presumed infectious until proven otherwise. Cases should be monitored and staff should be aware if the patient is a suspected case, probable case, or confirmed case of the disease. A suspected case is a patient that presents with clinical presentation of a disease, but no laboratory data is available. A probable case has clinical symptoms and can be directly linked to a confirmed case or has some preliminary laboratory evidence that the disease is present. Confirmed cases have definitive data; some confirmed cases may not have clinical manifestations. Staff should also monitor all wounds carefully for infections, particularly after disasters because of the risk of developing multi-drug resistant infections. Stockpiles of treatment items for endemic diseases should be created with instructions (and be on hand) for use.

14.7. UNTRAINED VOLUNTEERS

In many disaster situations, organizations will send volunteers that have no medical training, and members of the stricken community often want to help those in need. Untrained volunteers may become vectors for disease transmission and become ill themselves if some training in basic infection control principals is not completed prior to deployment. This is particularly important when the volunteers will be assisting medical personnel. The paramount importance of hand hygiene should be stressed, as well as the importance of good personal hygiene and sanitation practices. Beliefs about disease and traditional health practices for the area should be assessed and incorporated into care to improve compliance with hygiene and sanitation. When traditional health beliefs conflict with infection control methodologies, time should be taken to explain why following recommendations will help preserve human life in the current disaster situation. Additionally, subcontractors that provide services like housekeeping and food preparation may not have exposure to infection control methodologies and have potential to cause great harm if they are not briefed on prevention methods prior to providing services (Vane *et al.*, 2010).

14.8. INTERPRETATION/APPLICATION OF INFECTION CONTROL DATA

The team Joan is working with also receives patients from a different disaster facility . . . Her newest patient arrives . . . he has a persistent dry cough, diminished breath sounds, and fever. The patient denies having asthma or respiratory issues. He states he has had a cough for a few months and sometimes wakes up in a cold sweat. Joan consults with the medical personnel from the sending facility and . . . not taken a chest radiograph because it was unavailable and his laboratory values were consistent with what you would expect in trauma patients.

In disaster situations, access to laboratory and radiologic diagnostics may not be available or be extremely limited. Practitioners should be briefed on diseases endemic to the area, particularly those capable of causing outbreaks. In our case study, TB is endemic to the area and the patient presented with clinical symptoms of the disease. Providers should have excellent clinical skills, since supporting data for diagnosis may not be available. The close quarters and limited resources in mobile health units result in an environment ripe for spread of disease if practitioners are not vigilant about performing infection control measures and identifying potentially infectious patients early.

14.9. PATIENT SAFETY AND HEALTH SYSTEM ISSUES

In disaster situations, multiple agencies may send teams to provide care for those affected. It is important for one organization to take the lead in coordinating services offered at each location to optimize use of limited resources. The severity of the disaster will usually determine what agency is in control of coordinating relief efforts to the area. In the United States, the federal government is responsible for coordinating the response to high level disasters and utilizes the National Incident Management System (NIMS) to aid recovery and limit damage and death in the affected area (Izenberg, 2006). The NIMS is a general framework that is utilized in disasters to coordinate efforts between national, local, and volunteer agencies in a standardized manner. In less severe incidents, the local authority will coordinate efforts. To minimize redundancy and maximize resources, organizations should be made aware of the coordinating agency and what services are being provided by other agencies.

An example of coordinated relief efforts and how it relates to infection control is exemplified by the disaster response to the earthquake in Haiti in 2010. The Israeli Defense Forces Medical Corps, University of Miami, and the Red Cross coordinated efforts to care for patients devastated by the earthquake (Kreiss *et al.*, 2010). The Israeli Medical Corps was the first unit to arrive after the earthquake stuck. They brought personnel and facilities with the ability to perform surgical procedures, and had limited laboratory and imaging capabilities. When the University of Miami arrived and built facilities that initially did not have the same capabilities, they would take less acute patients and some patients from the Israeli Medical Corps facility post operatively. This transfer of patients allowed the Corps to perform needed surgical procedures on patients in need and the University continued care post-operatively to minimize complications and ensure that the necessary care was being provided. This allowed for life and limb saving surgeries; however, it added additional risks for spreading infections between facilities. From the published literature, it is unclear what precautions were taken for patients being transferred between facilities. Additionally, patients may be transferred to medical facilities outside of the disaster area.

During this particular episode, patients were transferred to neighboring countries that could offer specialized inpatient care. When patients are transferred to acute care settings outside the disaster zone, it is recommended that the patient be actively screened for infection. Incoming patients from flooding disasters should be placed on contact isolation, and not cohorted, because they carry the risk of being infected with various multi-drug resistant gram-negative bacteria. For the same reason, empiric antibiotic treatment should be avoided if an infection is suspected until culture results are obtained. If infections develop many weeks after the disaster and the illness is life-threatening, antibiotics for non-fermenting bacteria should be prescribed (Uckay *et al.*, 2006). Patients should also be placed on isolation if they are being admitted from a known outbreak area.

During the disaster in Haiti, there was an outbreak of Cholera. When an outbreak of a communicable disease occurs during disasters, a number of steps should be taken. Identification and confirmation of the infectious agent is required as soon as laboratory resources are available. Samples should be collected prior to administration of antibiotics or other treatment agents. Treatment should not be withheld if laboratory access is not immediately available, but all attempts should be made to acquire samples that will remain viable whenever possible. Most biologic samples will remain viable up to 24 hours at room temperature and many remain viable for up to 2 days if held at 4–8°C, with the exception of cold sensitive agents like meningococcus. Serum that is used for disease identification by detecting antibodies can usually be stored up to 10 days at 4–8°C. It may be possible to obtain results from antibody testing from samples held for a number of weeks at room temperature (Connolly, 2005) Therefore, if refrigeration is not immediately available, samples should still be acquired and held until laboratory confirmation is possible.

In the event there is an epidemic, an outbreak control team should be established. The team will be responsible for investigating and monitoring the outbreak to determine the extent and severity of the outbreak. Based on information obtained during the investigation, the team should determine the source of the outbreak, identify route of transmission, and develop prevention and treatment protocols. They should establish a control plan with the main goals of preventing exposure, infection, disease, and death. For example, if there were an outbreak of Malaria at the emergency mobile health unit you were stationed in your goals would be to kill mosquitoes (prevent exposure), provide mosquito nets and DEET insecticide (prevent infection), provide chemoprophylaxis for those at high risk (prevent disease), and identify and treat cases promptly (prevent death). In disaster situations, patient isolation is rarely feasible, or desired, with the exception of severe diseases like viral hemorrhagic fevers (Connolly, 2005).

14.10. SUMMARY POINTS

- Sanitation issues related to lack of suitable waste management facilities and adequate water are main contributors to the spread of disease in disaster situations
- Corpses who perish from trauma pose little threat of spreading disease, those that die of infectious diseases must follow additional protocols
- Instrument sterilization can be completed with bleach and alcohol baths
- Vector borne illnesses are likely and precautions should be taken to control them
- Efforts should be made to control crowding and to educate patients and family on sanitation and hygiene in disaster situations
- Transfer of disaster victims poses a threat for widespread disease transfer

14.11. REFERENCES

Chu, K.M., Trelles, M. and Ford, N.P. (2011). Quality of care in humanitarian surgery. *World Journal of Surgery, 35*(6): 1169–74. doi:10.1007/s00268-011-1084-9

Connolly, M.A. (2005). Communicable Disease Control in Emergencies: A Field Manual. No. (WHO/CDS/2005.27) World Health Organization.

Cruz, A.T., Patel, B., DiStefano, M.C., *et al.* (2010). Outside the box and into thick air: Implementation of an exterior mobile pediatric emergency response team for North American H1N1 (swine) influenza virus in Houston, Texas. *Annals of Emergency Medicine, 55*(1): 23–31. doi:10.1016/j.annemergmed.2009.08.003

Isenberg, S. (2006). Civilian application of military resources. The Surgical Clinics of North America, 86(3): 665–673. doi:10.1016/j.suc.2006.03.003

Kreiss, Y., Merin, O., Pele, K., *et al.* (2010). Early disaster response in Haiti: The Israeli field hospital experience. *Annals of Internal Medicine, 153*(1): 45-W.26. Retrieved from http://ezproxy.library.und.edu/login?url=http://search.ebscohost.com/login.as px?direct=true&db=aph&AN=52103729&site=ehost-live&scope=site

Lichtenberger, P., Masking, I.N., Dickinson, G., *et al.* (2010). Infection control in field hospitals after a natural disaster: Lessons learned after the 2010 earthquake in Haiti. *Infection Control and Hospital Epidemiology: The Official Journal of the Society of Hospital Epidemiologists of America, 31*(9): 951–957. doi:10.1086/656203

Noji, E.K. (2005). Public health issues in disasters. *Critical Care Medicine, 33*(1 Suppl): S29–33.

Rebmann, T., English, J.F. and Carrico, R. (2007). Disaster preparedness lessons learned and future directions for education: Results from focus groups conducted at the 2006 APIC conference. *American Journal of Infection Control, 35*(6): 374–381. doi: 10.1016/j.aijc.2006.09.002

Uckay, I., Sax, H., Harbarth, S., Bernard, L. and Pittet, D. (2008). Multi-resistant infections in repatriated patients after natural disasters: Lessons learned from the 2004 tsunami for hospital infection control. *Journal of Hospital Infection, 68*: 1–8. doi: 10.1016/j.jhin2007.10.018

Vane, E.A., Winthrop, T.G. and Martinez, L.M. (2010). Implementing basic infection control practices in disaster situations. *Nursing Clinics of North America, 45*: 219–231. doi: 10.1016/j.cnur.2010.02.011

Wang, M.Y. (2010). Devastation after the Haiti earthquake: A neurosurgeon's journal. *World Neurosurgery, 73*: 438–441. doi: 10.1016/j.wneu.2010.03.040

Waring, S.C. and Brown, B.J. (2005). The threat of communicable diseases following natural disasters: A public health response. *Disaster Management & Response: DMR : An Official Publication of the Emergency Nurses Association, 3*(2): 41–47. doi:10.1016/j.dmr.2005.02.003

CHAPTER 15

Future Issues in Monitoring for Safe Infection Control Practices

DENISE M. KORNIEWICZ Ph.D., RN, FAAN

This final chapter will expose the user to future ideas related to monitoring, surveillance, accountability and reimbursements. Topics will include ideas associated with "safe" infection control patient environments, public awareness and patient advocacy.

15.1. CASE PRESENTATION

The year is 2025 and Susie is an infection preventionist working in one of the "smart" hospital environments that was developed to eradicate infections. Due to the regulations associated with patient safety and outcomes associated with "best practices", changes in the way infection prevention nurses function has been changed. As a result, all nurses working in this new role are now held accountable for their actions and often receive less pay if they cause a patient to have an infection based on their actions. For example, Susie had to learn new skills associated with the epidemiology of infection, monitoring, and surveillance and adhere to new protocols related to collecting infection control data. Additionally, she had to have several courses in computers, informatics and databases. As a result, Susie's new responsibilities include data collection methods, analysis and interpretation of data.

Inherent in their new job role, Susie has had to determine the knowledge of the patient or consumer because now the consumer had to complete educational modules prior to their admittance to the healthcare setting. In fact, the patient now has to not only provide the history, physician, and procedure, but they have to sign and note that they know the infection control data about the healthcare provider (HCP). For example, the institution as well

233

as data from other national institutions has readily provided the rate of infection associated with a surgical site infection by their HCP. Susie also is obligated to answer any questions the patient may have if they do not understand the information available. Susie is now required to document the educational level of the patient and the patients' ability to understand the procedure.

Susie reviews the computer as Mr. James comes in for admission. She brings with her "SAM", which is the "sensored avatar man". SAM provides instant video feed about Mr. James' blood work, preoperative teaching modules and a message from his physician. Additionally, SAM provides a simple comprehension test on Mr. James to assess his understanding of his procedure. Mr. James is intrigued by this new technology but is aware that this is an essential component of his pre-operative phase. Mr. James is instructed that a similar SAM will be available in the post-operative wing so that HCPs do not expose him to unwarranted bloodborne pathogens.

Mr. James is walked to the pre-operative "model" hospital room. He peers inside and notices that everything in the room is modern, blue-tooth connected, clean and very sophisticated. Susie instructs Mr. James about the use of high-tech equipment in the hospital environment and tells him that from the time he enters until he leaves, he will be continuously monitored for any type of infection, adverse event or any change in his well being. Mr. James is amazed at this new hospital environment but is pleased that all the necessary equipment will help him to stay healthy.

Last, Mr. James is instructed that he may bring a patient advocate to the healthcare setting. The patient advocate can be a family member or someone that is hired by Mr. James. The role of the patient advocate is to provide information to the healthcare team related to the continuity of his care, assist in communicating with a variety of healthcare providers and assisting Mr. James with his understanding of his hospitalization. Mr. James has never experienced a person in this role; however, he welcomes the patient advocate because he is not sure about the healthcare environment, equipment or all the different providers.

15.2. ESSENTIAL CONTENT INFECTION CONTROL OF THE FUTURE

Consumer awareness has been enhanced by the use of information that is available by the Internet. Today, consumers can access information related to their healthcare facility, healthcare provider, type of healthcare procedure, type of treatment available and types of medical devices used for diagnostic procedures. General principles associated with the future for controlling both community acquired or healthcare associated infections include methods that provide the information technology platforms that accurately monitor global or local infections. The consistent implementation of monitoring methods to eliminate healthcare associated infections, epidemics, emerging infections and prevent widespread non-compliance of infection control strategies requires consistent diligence to prevent consumers from widespread infections.

Susie had to learn new skills associated with the epidemiology of infection, monitoring, surveillance and adhere to new protocols related to collecting infection control data. Additionally, she had to have several courses in computers, informatics and databases. As a result, Susie's new responsibilities include data collection methods, analysis and interpretation of data.

15.2.1. Monitoring and Surveillance Measures

The most effective infection control methods include the monitoring of impending infections and alerts that prompt healthcare providers (HCPs) to intervene early. Surveillance programs that are based on sound epidemiological principles that include protection for the patient population, HCPs and the environment have demonstrated to be safe and cost-effective methods that reduce the rate of infections. Examples include surveillance of healthcare associated infections, antibiotic resistance patterns, monitoring of patient falls, medication errors, surgical site infections, medical device infections such as indwelling catheters, central line infections and HCPs' compliance to hand hygiene. Internal methods for monitoring adverse events associated with infection prevention may include the use of computer based systems that provide on-line feedback to the HCPs through computer linkages to the clinical laboratory reports and antibiotic treatments. Most recently, Wenzel (2010) has demonstrated that early changes with the use of antibiotics based on the availability of clinical microbiology data assures early treatment interventions and reduces the length of stay for patients. Additionally, early detection for infection control patterns can be readily monitored and prevent infectious outbreak.

External surveillance for patterns of infections allows HCPs to benchmark or compare their rates of infection to other institutions. For example, the rate of an infection may be linked to the patient population, the type of procedure, factors associated with safety practices or policies, patient risk factors or severity of illness, as well as the institutional infection control standards. Today, hospital administrators provide infection control data about specific procedures to the consumer. As a result, there has been a decrease in the number of healthcare acquired infections because of the sharing of data and an increased awareness among HCPs to intervene earlier (Pyrek, 2012).

15.2.2. Accountability Indicators

All healthcare organizations are subject to regulation and oversight by a variety of agencies or governing bodies to be accountable for both the safety of patients and HCPs. Often, infection control personnel assist with the data management associated with the institution's compliance to the legislated mandates. These include employee health requirements such as inoculation against communicable diseases (TB, influenza, etc.), as well as occupational health requirements related to health and safety education. The prevention of healthcare associated infections is dependent on the training and education of HCPs within the institution. Ongoing programs related to the knowledge and safety of patients as well as the reinforcement of policies provides the platform for successful accountability.

Most recently, the use of video monitoring and feedback programs that demonstrate compliance or the lack of compliance in the adherence to infection control standards has assisted HCPs to decrease the rate of HAIs in hospital settings (Smith, 2006). Training techniques that incorporate active observance of HCP behavior has encouraged participation by HCPs to be proactive to increase hand hygiene compliance. Additionally, the use of tracking devices that remind HCPs to wash their hands has assisted in the development of new policies that foster increased accountability among all HCPs.

On the national level, new policies associated with Medicare and Medicaid reimbursement surrounding healthcare associated infections has sought to hold institutions and or providers accountable for the provision and actions of the care they have rendered. Specific tracking of HCPs via video devices, RFDs and room to room monitoring has captured data about HCP behaviors related to "how" care is provided, whether or not infection control procedures have been followed and if the HCP has been compliant to safe patient care. These monitoring systems have been instituted at some institutions; however, accountability policies and procedures for HCPs continues to be developed (Schatz *et al.*, 2012).

15.2.3. Reimbursement Factors

A number of reimbursement initiatives associated with patient safety and the rate of reimbursement for patients who acquire an infection during hospitalization has awakened healthcare administrators to improve computer technology platforms that accurately track infections among patients. Most importantly, infection control preventionists have had to develop new policies and guidelines that hold HCPs accountable for their care. For example, Swoboda *et al.* (2007) demonstrated that the use of electronic monitoring and voice command improved hand hygiene compliance among HCPs and decreased the rates of healthcare associated infections. New tracking devices that provide immediate feedback to HCPs may assist in decreasing the overall cost of healthcare associated infections by actively reminding HCPs to be compliant to factors associated with good hand hygiene techniques.

15.3. FUTURE ENGINEERING CONTROLS

Advancements in the use of engineering controls that can automatically monitor infection control practices in both community or healthcare settings will provide data that may reduce the overall cost of healthcare. Specific changes may include simple to complex re-engineered medical devices. For example, the adaptation of the use of "barcodes" or radio frequency sensors (RFID) to track medical equipment and instruments provides additional safety in the operating room since all instruments can be scanned before and after a surgical case. An additional feature such as the use of an "infrared" technique can add to the identification of a contaminated instrument, thus eliminating the possible risk of an infection for a surgical patient.

The use of HCP nametags that use RFID sensors to monitor when HCPs enter, leave, and use hand-hygiene equipment while sensing and monitoring activity provides increased compliance among HCPs during patient care activities. RFID systems are not new; however, the application to the healthcare environment may prove to be beneficial by providing immediate feedback to HCPs. Additionally, the use of RFID systems can also be used to tag equipment so that monitors, IV poles, glucometers, beds, telemetry devices or computers can be tracked throughout the patient environment. This would provide easy access to HCPs so that contaminated or unsafe patient care equipment could be removed from the patient's immediate environment.

> She brings with her "SAM" which is the "sensored avatar man". SAM provides instant video feed about Mr. James's blood work, preoperative teaching modules and a message from his physician. Additionally, SAM provides a simple comprehension test on Mr. James to assess his understanding of his procedure. Mr. James is intrigued by this new technology but is aware that this is an essential component of his pre-operative phase.

The use of robots with video applications that can move from patient to patient making rounds without the HCP "touching" the patient can decrease cross contamination between patients. Embedded within the robotic features would be the ability to monitor the patient's vital signs and the ability to scan the environment, integrate with the electronic health record as well as provide educational information for the patient or HCP. Use of a "smart" robotic video platform that provides two-way communication (verbal or written) gives immediate feedback to the patient and HCP. Additionally, these personal care robots may have adaptable features that provide both the patient and HCP with the ability to communicate with each other.

The addition of auto-tracking video cameras with computerized data interfaces would allow for analysis of infection control events. The technology platforms already exist with hand-held devices; however, the addition of video cameras with integrated motion sensors would be a feature that would provide data associated with "in time" infection control practices.

The use of environmental monitoring cleaning technology platforms that allow for misting the environment to decrease environmental contaminants has been developed (Seil, 2012). Other products associated with the use of nanotechnology particles that automatically clean surfaces and decrease microbial bioburden may be enhanced features for infection prevention environments. Use of fabrics for patient care or HCP protection that provides an "end of life" use for infection protection may be products of the future that are used in healthcare environments to decrease environmental contaminants.

15.4. SAFETY THROUGH KNOWLEDGE

The Centers for Disease Control & Prevention has assisted in educating the public about the importance of infection control practices as a factor of patient safety. Specifically, individuals who acquire a healthcare-associated infection (HAI) are patients who acquire an infection as a result of receiving healthcare treatment for other conditions. HAIs can be deadly and the best way to prevent these infections is to provide preventive measures that impact on the patient, environment and the HCP. Initiatives such as "Speak Up," "Keeping Your Hands Clean," and "Asking Your Healthcare Provider" are patient safety educational modules offered by the CDC (2012). Therefore, one of the best ways to provide safer patient environments is to empower patients through education, use of new and safer medical devices and provide feedback loops consistent with tracking infections.

Susie has had to determine the knowledge of the patient or consumer because now the consumer has to complete educational modules prior to their admittance to the healthcare setting. In fact, the patient now has to not only provide the history, physician and procedure, but they have to sign and note that they know the infection control data about the healthcare provider (HCP).

Healthcare knowledge among patients or providers can be transformative to achieve increased patient safety, quality, team, and patient-centered or cost-effective care. It is the use of strategic processes that include a concerted, systematic approach to identifying the interplay among healthcare disciplines and actions of the HCPs that contribute to clinical decision making for good patient outcomes. Safety through knowledge includes tracking data associated with the patient, provider, resources and healthcare environment available. As a result, new methods that are in the process of development include the interplay between human factors, technology, virtual networks, and the overall general environmental improvements to provide safer patient care.

15.4.1. Integration of Technology and Human Factors

Human factors include the investigation of how the environment, organization and job factors, and human and individual characteristics influence behavior in the workplace. Additionally, human factors include any issue that can affect the health and safety of an individual. Human factors include three major aspects: the job, the individual and the organization and how they impact people's health and safety-related behavior. Infection control practices can readily adapt the principles of human factors by applying the interaction between the HCP, the design of medical devices and the system in which they perform. Studying the interaction related to infection prevention techniques, feedback mechanisms for HCPs, workload, ergonomic design and general workplace environments can be used to increase compliance with practices to prevent hospital-acquired infections. Examples include studies associated with compliance to hand hygiene by using RFID tags or sensors to find the equipment for cleaning one's hands in a busy clinical environment (Schweon *et al.*, 2012). HCPs can now be instantly reminded by a voice command or signal to remind them to clean their hands prior to touching a patient.

Other human factor initiatives include the systematic application of evidence-based interventions that have been demonstrated to reduce the risk of HAIs. Since most HCPs have to recall thousands of pieces of information in a normal working day, the use of automated systems that provide "alerts" to HCPs assist in the overall reduction of errors or adverse events. Human factor designs associated with the proper angle for intubated patients, re-engineering of the airway tube or an automatically designed bed that senses position may be future platforms that will be used in the clinical setting.

15.4.2. Automated Global Networks for Infection Control Surveillance

The development of inter-connected local, regional, national and global infection control surveillance programs are not new. What is new is the ability to transfer data from one system to the other in a matter of a short period of time. The CDC has developed a global laboratory network to identify invasive organisms and match treatment modalities. The use of "in-time" computer tracking devices such as these will encourage HCP at the bedside to access these information systems to provide immediate treatment. Examples of these networks include National Nosocomial Infection Surveillance system (NNIS), which obtains global data from intensive care units to track HAIs (CDC, 2012). Data that is collected includes the name, medical record, age, gender, underlying diseases, and severity of illness score at time of entrance to the ICU. Other data associated with temperature, blood pressure, use of invasive devices, cultures taken, presence of clinical pneumonia, antibiotic use, and characteristics of any infection is collected both for cases and controls daily. This allows analysis of cases and controls in prospective cohort nested studies.

These databanks provide data for studies that can modify the risk factors associated with invasive devices (Infection Control, 2012). Surveillance can lead to an understanding of the causality related to HAIs and result in more effective and targeted interventions. Data related to performance feedback on hand hygiene compliance, vascular catheter or Foley care, mechanical ventilation and surgical site infections have showed a reduction in HAI rates, decreased mortality, decreased length of stay and cost associated with antibiotic use. Currently, HCPs are able to obtain national benchmarks associated with HAIs; however, in the future, the databases and computer networking systems will be modified to encompass "in-time" data. This will allow for HCPs to make clinical treatment decisions at the bedside versus waiting for results or comparative data.

Mr. James is walked to the pre-operative "model" hospital room. He peers inside and notices that everything in the room is modern, blue-tooth connected, clean and very sophisticated. Susie instructs Mr. James about the use of high-tech equipment in the hospital environment and tells him that from the time he enters until he leaves, he will be continuously monitored for any type of infection, adverse event or any change in his well being.

15.4.3. Environmental Monitoring

The ability to control the healthcare environment to make it "infection free" may be the next architectural development for future hospitals. The use of a "smart" technology incorporating sensors within the environment as well as embedded in clothing of the HCP may be the environment of the future. For example, the ability to obtain error-proof systems or processes that actively identify real-time information about an impending infection can assist in the overall prevention of an infection. Use of nanotechnological mattresses, gowns, gloves or blankets may provide a cleaner environment. The development of continuous cleaning for non-contaminated air or dirty vents may be a future required standard. A decontamination spray during "room" turnover may be incorporated in the future as well as the use of robots for cleaning versus human beings. All of these platforms of the future may have an initial cost however, through the prevention of secondary complications, super-infections or increased length of stay, patients will have better clinical outcomes and decreased adverse events.

15.5. FUTURE PATIENT PARTICIPATION, PUBLIC AWARENESS AND PATIENT ADVOCACY

The future for monitoring safe infection control practices is dependent on the symbiotic relationship between the patient and the HCP. The patient will be more knowledgeable about his or her own health prior to admission to a healthcare environment. At the same time, the HCP will be held accountable for their actions by being trained to provide data driven interventions. In order to be successful, the HCP will need to learn new skills that integrate the patient as an equal team member when providing patient care. The patient as an active participant and knowledgeable consumer will be new to most HCPs.

As patients become more and more familiar about healthcare reform issues and understand the concept of "benchmarking" one provider compared to another, increased public awareness will change the accountability of HCP and change the delivery of healthcare. Public awareness may assist in improving the current healthcare system while providing new ways for patients to access healthcare. Competition for healthcare providers may become a more level "playing field" since new government mandates will be expected. For example, a "no tolerance policy" associated with a HAI may be mandated and reimbursement will be not be allowed if the HAI occurred as a result of medical or nursing treatment. Additionally, HCPs may have to pay fines if their actions purposely caused an HAI. Therefore, as the consumer becomes more educated and public awareness becomes an expected norm, the outcomes associated with excellent patient care becomes more important.

Last, Mr. James is instructed that he may bring a patient advocate to the healthcare setting. The patient advocate can be a family member or someone that is hired by Mr. James. The role of the patient advocate is to provide information to the healthcare team related to the continuity of his care, assist in communicating with a variety of healthcare providers and assisting Mr. James with his understanding of his hospitalization.

In the future, new roles may develop for HCPs within the healthcare system. For example, the role of the infection control nurse has evolved to a new functional role called an infection preventionist. The new skills required of the infection preventionist require an understanding of informatics, data driven health models and the ability to use principles from multiple professional disciplines such as engineering, ethics, basic sciences, and the human sciences. New professional roles such as a professional patient advocate may evolve especially to coach patients through the healthcare delivery system. Patient advocates will be educated to navigate the patient through their healthcare event. This new role will provide patients with an additional resource to help them further understand their healthcare issue. Patient advocates may or may not be welcomed as part of the healthcare system because some HCPs may view this new role as competitive, since the patient will employ them. Their role will be to keep the patient informed, assist with healthcare decisions and provide easier transitions for the patients while receiving care.

The success of the future way we monitor HAIs and provide cost-effective care is dependent on what structures are federally mandated for reimbursement. At the national level, HCPs will have no choice to but to improve patient outcomes and decrease the rate of HAIs since reimbursement models will be based on data that demonstrates treatment modalities. For the healthcare environment, new methods that require HCPs to be accountable at the bedside will become an expected behavior and patients may rate HCPs. The feedback mechanism from evaluations by patients or other HCPs will require computer based systems that send data immediately to HCP so that they can immediately intervene. It will be the sophistication of these computer driven systems that will enhance the overall quality of healthcare.

15.6. SUMMARY POINTS

- Monitoring and surveillance measures will increase to provide data associated with HAIs
- Accountability in the future will include the HCP, the healthcare environment and reimbursement
- Future engineering controls will include the patient, HCP, equipment, use of robots, increased computerized data systems and environmental monitoring
- The use of human factors engineering will improve HAI outcomes
- The integration of global networks to monitor HAI will be available to clinicians

- Monitoring the environment and using newly designed materials will decrease the rate of HAIs
- Patients will be more knowledgeable and new roles will emerge related to patient advocacy

15.7. REFERENCES

Healthcare Associated Infections. http://www.cdc.gov/hai/ accessed 7/6/12

Patient Safety: Ten Things You Can Do to Be a Safe Patient. http://www.cdc.gov/HAI/ patientSafety/patient-safety.html accessed 6/27/12.

Pyrek, K. (2012). Trends in infection prevention and control experts share perspectives on key issues. Infectioncontroltoday.com/articles/2011/01/trends-infect (accessed 6/28/12).

Schweon, S.J., Edmonds, S.L., Kirk, J., Rowland, D.Y. and Acosta, C. (2012). Effectiveness of a comprehensive hand hygiene program for reduction of infection rates in a long-term care facility. *Am. J. Infect. Control.,* Jun 30.

Seil, J.T. and Webster, T.J. (2012). Antimicrobial applications of nanotechnology: methods and literature. *Int. J. Nanomedicine, 7*: 2767–81.

Smith, S.L. (2006). Do you think you have what it takes to set up a long-term video monitoring unit? *Am. J. Electroneurodiagnostic Technol., 46*(1): 49–55.

Society for Healthcare Epidemiology of America (SHEA), the Infectious Diseases Society of America (IDSA), and the Pediatric Infectious Diseases Society (PIDS). (2012). Policy statement on antimicrobial stewardship. *Infect. Control Hosp. Epidemiol., 33*(4):322–7.

Swoboda, S.M., Earsing, K., Strauss, K., Lane, S. and Lipsett, P.A. (2007). Isolation status and voice prompts improve hand hygiene. (2007). *Am. J. Infect. Control, 35*(7): 470–6.

Vallejos, S.C.H., Medeiros, H.P., Schneider, F.K. and Abatti, P.J. (2012). Wireless medical sensor networks: design requirements and enabling technologies. *Telemed. J. E. Health, 18*(5): 394-9. Epub 2012 Apr 13.

Wenzel, R.P. (2010) Minimizing surgical-site infections. *N. Engl. J. Med., 362*(1): 75–7.

Index

Accountability, 1, 9, 10, 15, 132, 192, 233, 236, 237, 242, 243

acinetobactor spp, 74

Adherence, 5, 15, 29, 30, 32, 76, 83, 87, 105, 116, 136, 145, 160, 184, 195, 196, 201, 209, 236

advanced practice nurses, 5, 14, 44, 90, 175

Airborne, 34, 38, 38, 80, 82, 83, 84, 86, 114, 134, 209, 221

alcohol-based hand rub, 40

Ambulatory, 111, 121, 192, 203

antibiotic-resistant bacteria, 35, 123

Antibiotics, 2, 36, 44, 87, 88, 96, 97, 105, 117, 123, 145, 209, 210, 229, 235

antimicrobial soap, 40, 76, 77, 137

Antisepsis, 8, 76, 190, 194, 197, 203

bacillus anthracis, 77

Bactericidal, 133

barrier precautions, 8, 46, 89, 96–98, 104, 107

Behavioral, 7, 14, 29, 40, 45, 46, 174, 175, 177, 186, 187

best practice, 13, 14, 32

Biochemical, 109, 117, 118, 121

bloodborne pathogens, 19, 21, 22, 26–28, 78, 80–83, 96, 115, 197, 234

body fluids, 21, 22, 24, 76, 77, 80, 83, 96, 116, 119, 147, 162, 181, 198

catheter-related, 17, 39, 92, 98, 107, 108

Centers for Medicare and Medicaid Services, 4, 16, 203

Centers for Disease Control, 196

central line infections, 98, 235

chain of infection, 33, 35, 37, 39, 41, 43, 45, 47, 133–135, 183

Chlorhexidine, 3, 8, 13, 66, 75, 77, 99, 101–107, 151, 196, 197, 203

Chronic, 91, 143, 150, 111

CLABSI, 2–8, 10, 99, 101–105, 107

Cleanliness, 47, 160, 161, 180, 200, 200

clinical environment, 14, 240

clostridium difficile, 74, 91, 117, 120, 125, 127, 130, 151, 155, 156, 180, 188, 205, 211, 213

Clothing, 24, 31, 38, 42, 43, 72, 74, 145, 161, 162, 176, 181, 210, 222, 241

Collaboration, 14, 88

Colonization, 34–37, 42, 89, 146, 150, 151, 181

Communicable, 33, 69, 89, 90, 141, 145, 149, 150, 171, 174, 185, 192, 200, 205, 212, 215, 222, 225, 229, 231, 236

Communication, 8, 11, 14, 150, 158, 160, 166, 223, 226, 238

Community, 41, 49, 55, 120, 139, 202, 206, 210, 213

Community acquired infections, 1, 205

co-morbidities, 150

Compliance, 2, 3, 6, 7, 9–11, 13, 16, 26, 39–42, 44–46, 76, 77, 81–83, 88, 91, 92–94, 96, 98, 99, 107, 146, 168, 179, 185, 192, 199, 213, 223, 227, 235–237, 240, 241

confidence intervals, 50, 61, 63, 67

245

Consumer, 4, 15, 146, 233–236, 242
Contagious, 109, 117, 181, 210
Contamination, 24, 40, 42, 43, 45, 47,
    48, 77, 84, 89, 104, 109, 120, 123,
    125, 134, 135, 137, 141, 143, 148,
    161, 162, 178, 183, 194, 197, 200,
    207, 215, 218–220, 225, 238
cost-effective, 1, 9, 155, 210, 235, 239
Culture, 1, 3, 5, 8, 10, 14, 15, 21, 22,
    27–30, 35, 43, 44, 46, 86, 96, 97,
    99, 101, 123, 131–133, 135, 137,
    139, 148–150, 219, 229
cumulative incidence, 49, 50, 51, 53, 67

Data, 9, 11, 14–18, 21, 23–26, 30, 41, 44,
    49, 50, 51, 53, 55, 57, 61, 63–65,
    67, 73, 76, 82, 83, 92, 95, 97, 98,
    101–103, 105, 124, 141, 150, 165,
    167, 185, 197, 198, 212, 217, 220,
    227, 228, 233–243
Density, 52
Detection, 17, 48, 108, 183, 206, 235
Diagnosis, 51, 86, 89, 90, 109, 111, 114,
    115, 126, 145, 177, 182, 185, 211,
    228
direct contact, 37, 40, 145
Disaster, 117, 123, 124, 216–220,
    223–231
disease frequency, 50, 54, 67
Disinfect, 27, 118, 137, 223
Disposable, 130, 147, 163, 194

Economic, 4, 9, 15, 16, 108, 198
Education, 5, 14, 25, 27–32, 40, 43,
    44, 77, 85, 88, 101, 104, 106, 141,
    142, 146, 151, 152, 159, 166, 167,
    185–187, 198, 205–207, 211, 212,
    231, 236, 239
Electronic, 80, 96, 98, 121, 155, 237, 238
electronic health records (E H R), 80
Endogenous, 37, 44, 45, 88, 134
engineering controls, 69, 78, 79–81, 92,
    94, 237, 243
environmental flora, 35
Epidemic, 126, 133, 216, 218, 221
Epidemiology, 5, 17, 31, 32, 36, 47,
    50, 55, 67, 90, 92, 107, 125, 126,
    133, 139, 155, 156, 165, 187, 198,
    201–213, 231, 235, 244

evidence-based standards, 5
evidenced-based practices, 8
Exogenous, 45, 88, 134
Exposure, 20, 22, 23, 25–28, 35–37, 42,
    50, 55–60, 63, 67, 80–82, 88, 96,
    97, 114, 116, 118, 121, 124–126,
    171, 185, 186, 210, 226, 230

Food, 65, 136–139, 173–180, 206–212,
    223, 227
food safety, 177, 187, 206, 213, 223

Gloves, 47, 48, 72, 74, 76, 77, 82, 84,
    92, 96–98, 106, 115, 130, 133, 145,
    147, 152, 179, 181, 193, 198, 223,
    241
Guidelines, 5–8, 16, 19, 20, 26, 30, 31,
    39–42, 47, 67, 75–77, 82, 83, 85,
    87, 89, 91, 92, 94, 107, 115, 125,
    131, 136, 138, 139, 141–146, 148,
    153–156, 166, 167, 178, 184–187,
    189–192, 195, 199, 201, 212, 237

hand hygiene, 2, 3, 6, 8, 9, 11, 26, 34,
    39, 40, 42, 44–47, 69, 73, 75–77,
    82, 83, 87–89, 92–94, 96–98, 113,
    116, 117, 137, 145–148, 151, 153,
    565–158, 161, 164, 168, 181, 182,
    184, 185, 187, 190, 210, 212, 216,
    218, 219, 223, 227, 235, 237, 240,
    241, 244
hazard ratio, 55, 58, 63, 64, 67
Healthcare associated infections, 16, 46,
    92, 116, 162
high risk, 39, 41, 114, 138, 160, 163,
    178, 230
home health, 157–160, 162–164,
    166–168
human factors, 239, 240, 243
human reservoirs, 37, 46

Immunity, 134, 208, 213, 216
Immunization, 49, 157, 206, 208, 223,
    200
Immunosuppression, 36
Implant, 143
Improvement, 2, 4, 6, 8, 11, 13, 15, 16,
    26, 29, 30–32, 40, 91, 98, 117

inanimate objects, 74, 117, 134, 138, 161
indirect contact, 37, 38, 84, 88
infection control, 1–16, 17, 19, 20–246
infection preventionist, 13, 90, 200, 233, 243
infectious disease, 20, 21, 29, 33, 37, 91, 92, 107, 109, 111, 112, 119–122, 132, 137, 150, 168, 185, 203, 206, 208, 209, 213, 224
Infrastructure, 8, 17, 135, 212, 218
Institute of Medicine, 18
Institutional, 2, 125, 175, 181, 236
intensive care, 2, 16, 33, 38, 39, 46, 47, 70, 73, 77, 86, 87, 88, 92, 93, 95, 99, 100, 107, 108, 197, 203, 226, 240
Intravenous, 13, 20, 22, 28, 33, 42, 96, 97, 101, 104, 110, 115, 120, 157, 165
Isolation, 24, 33–35, 37–39, 41, 43–45, 47, 69, 70, 71, 73, 82–85, 87–89, 91–94, 111, 112, 114–118, 121, 122, 126, 148, 152, 174, 182–184, 217, 221, 227, 229, 230, 244

latex, 20, 23, 24, 26, 31, 32, 92
Legal, 3, 19, 20, 29, 30
long-term care, 141, 147, 155, 244

Magnet hospital, 1
medical devices, 35, 79, 81, 136–139, 166, 235, 239, 240
mental health, 171–185
methicillin-resistant S. aureus, 34, 35
Microorganisms, 22, 33, 37, 38, 73, 76, 125, 130, 131, 133–135, 137, 145, 148, 152, 161, 163, 196, 197
Mobility, 121, 182, 187, 217
Monitoring, 6, 9, 29, 40, 44, 69, 80, 83, 87, 89, 120, 129, 132, 135, 144, 153, 176, 186, 194, 198, 199, 210, 211, 230, 233, 235–237
Morbidity, 4, 12, 73, 74, 76, 87, 88, 92, 211, 215
Mortality, 4, 12, 54, 55, 73, 74, 76, 77, 88, 92, 99, 211, 215, 221, 241
multidisciplinary team, 5
multi-drug resistant organism, 5, 41

National Healthcare Safety Network, 4
National Institute of Occupational Safety and Health, 20
needle stick injuries, 19, 31
Networks, 239, 240, 243, 244
Noncompliant, 3, 9
Norovirus, 74, 94, 116, 120, 127, 187, 188
nurse staffing, 35, 38, 39, 47
nursing rounds, 102–105

Occupational Safety and Health Administration (OSHA), 81
odds ratio, 59, 60, 63, 64, 67, 98
operating room, 13, 19, 71, 190, 193, 200, 237
Outbreak, 38, 47, 49, 75, 89, 112, 117, 118, 122, 124, 142, 144, 152, 171, 173, 177, 179, 183, 184, 191, 212, 223, 229, 230, 235
Overcrowding, 35, 39, 46, 47, 122, 217, 224, 226

Pathogenic, 37, 40, 42, 43, 45, 116, 125, 131, 146, 150, 161, 162, 176, 182, 196
patient advocacy, 233, 242, 244
Patient safety, 1, 8, 10, 14–16, 21, 23, 26, 29, 32, 33, 35, 37, 39, 40, 31, 43, 45–47, 73, 74, 90, 144, 153, 154, 156, 160, 166, 167, 175, 189, 192, 200, 212, 228, 233, 237, 239, 244
patient-centered, 131, 132
performance improvement, 4, 11, 12, 15
personal protective equipment, 19, 20, 22, 23, 26, 31, 78–80, 82, 91, 94, 115, 118, 133, 135, 147, 153, 162, 174, 182, 183
Practitioner, 1, 32, 33, 43, 50, 89–91, 95, 98, 100, 101, 129, 171, 202, 215
Prevalence, 53, 54
Prevention, 5–8, 11, 12, 14, 28, 29, 31, 39, 44, 81, 106–108, 130, 142, 167, 185, 208
Probability, 50, 55, 60, 61, 67, 72, 182
Procedure, 3, 7, 11, 12, 22, 24, 38, 46, 77, 82, 91, 98, 102, 106, 129, 133, 149, 189, 190, 193, 195, 197, 201, 202, 217, 233–236, 238, 239

process measure, 1, 9, 10, 15, 132, 192,
    233, 236, 237, 242, 243
Psychiatric, 171–188

Quality, 1–9, 11–14, 16, 17, 21, 26, 27,
    29–32, 39, 43, 53, 92, 101–102, 95,
    98, 111, 115, 118, 132, 137, 139,
    144, 163, 186, 199, 201, 202, 231,
    239, 243
quality metrics, 1, 11

radio frequency sensors, 237
Readiness, 7
relative risk, 50, 55–64, 66, 67
Respiratory, 25, 37, 38, 42, 44, 79,
    83–85, 111, 112, 114, 116, 119,
    121, 124, 126, 138, 144, 145, 148,
    154, 168, 177, 181, 185, 186, 217,
    221, 226, 228
Restraints, 184, 185
Reusable, 41, 43, 118, 120, 125, 126,
    136, 137, 139, 148, 202
Risk, 25–29, 32, 34–36, 39, 41, 44,
    49–52, 55–64, 66, 67, 78, 84–88,
    96–99, 114–116, 119, 122–126,
    129, 130, 132, 133, 137, 138, 143,
    146, 191–193, 196, 197, 200, 211,
    212, 218, 241
risk management, 3, 21, 26, 32, 126
role modeling, 14

Sanitation, 180, 186, 219, 227
Scrub, 101–106, 158, 193, 194, 200
Sensitivity, 86, 105
sharps injury, 27, 31, 79, 81, 82
Significance, 50, 62, 63, 66, 67, 209
Simulation, 82, 106
skin washes, 202
standard precautions, 20, 23, 40, 41, 44,
    72, 80, 83, 84, 113, 125, 144, 145,
    151, 167, 168, 197
staphylococcus aureus, 74, 94, 96, 116,
    120, 127, 187, 188

statistical tests, 61
Sterilization, 27, 135, 149, 230
surgical site infections, 4, 16, 17, 26,
    168, 198, 199, 235, 241, 244
Surveillance, 6, 10, 11, 23, 29, 30, 41,
    42, 51–54, 73, 83, 89, 90, 93, 101,
    106, 132, 144–146, 151, 153,
    167–169, 172, 179, 180, 185, 206,
    210, 211, 220, 221, 226, 233, 235,
    236, 240, 241, 243

Teamwork, 8, 9
Technology, 13, 27, 28, 81, 82, 88, 144,
    234, 245, 237–239, 241
Transmission, 22, 27, 29, 33, 37–45,
    83–88, 90, 92–94, 96, 97, 105,
    112, 113, 119, 121, 122, 124, 125,
    127, 129, 132–136, 139, 143, 146,
    150, 152, 154, 155, 161–168, 171,
    175, 177, 182, 183, 185, 189, 194,
    200–202, 205–213, 215, 221, 227,
    230
Trauma, 69, 71, 75, 88, 100, 118,
    119, 125, 215, 217, 220, 226,
    228, 230
Travel, 85, 117, 208, 226
Treatment, 36, 44, 45, 67, 72, 74, 88, 89,
    91, 110, 111, 113, 114, 116–119,
    123, 124, 133, 171, 172, 174, 177,
    183–185, 209, 210, 218, 227, 229,
    230, 235, 240–243
Tuberculosis, 111, 115, 236

Uncontrolled, 163, 166, 167, 213
universal precautions, 21, 81, 118
Unrestricted, 193

Vaccines, 87, 93, 116, 149, 154, 206,
    208, 209, 212, 213
vector borne, 218, 221, 222, 230
Video, 83, 234, 236, 238, 244

World Health Organization (WHO), 76